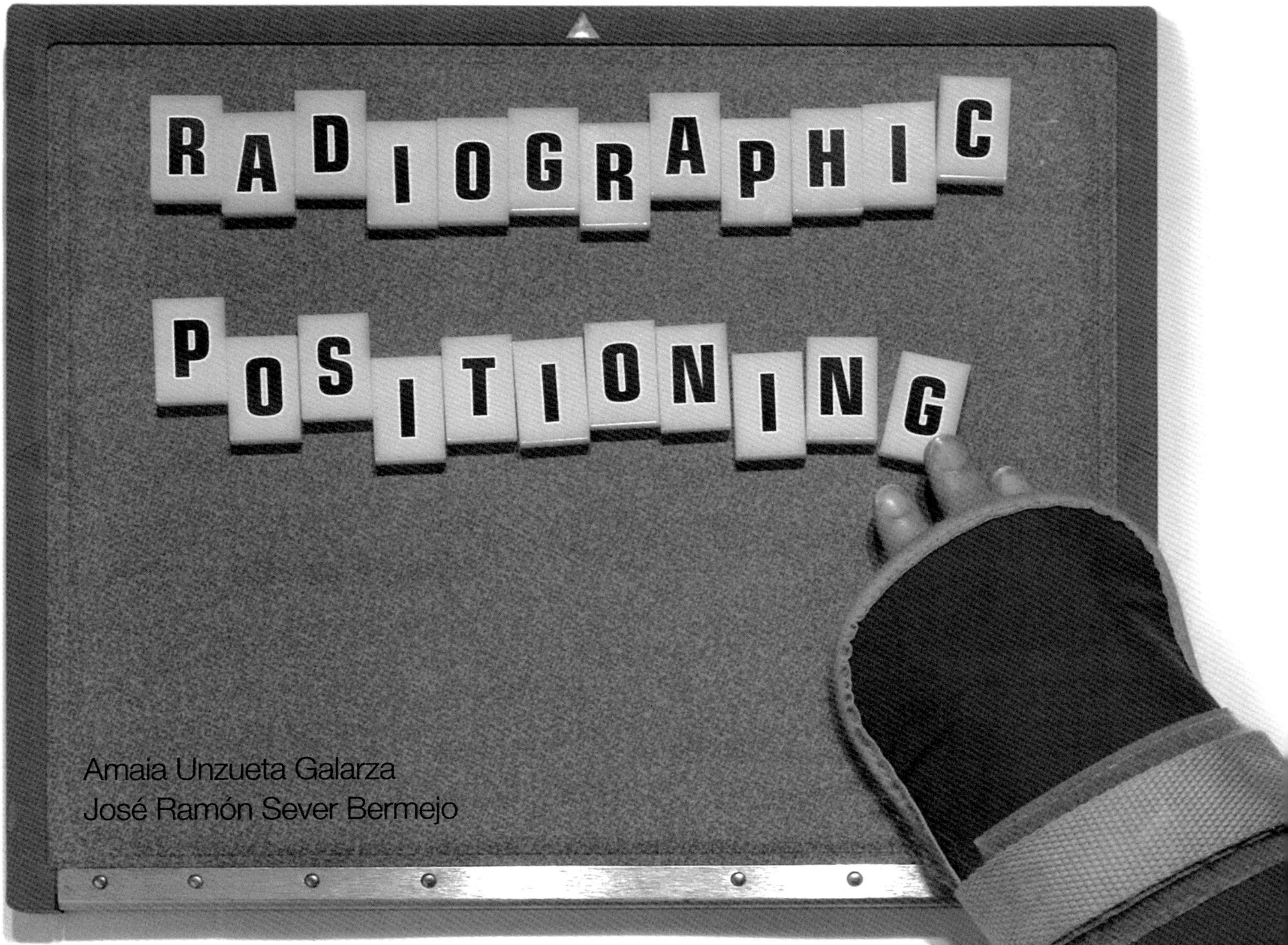

Amaia Unzueta Galarza
José Ramón Sever Bermejo

Handbook of radiographic positions and projections in the dog

Plaza Antonio Beltrán Martínez nº 1, planta 8 - letra I
(Centro empresarial El Trovador)
50002 Zaragoza - Spain

First printing: 2009

This book was originally published in Spanish under the title:
Manual de posiciones y proyecciones radiológicas en el perro
© 2008 Grupo Asís Biomedia, SL
ISBN Spanish edition: 978-84-935971-4-6

Translation/Proofreading:
Mette Bouman DVM
Ian Neville BVSc MRCVS
Karin de Lange, DVM MRCVS

ISBN: 978-84-92569-13-7
DL: NA-1777-2009

Design, layout and printing:
Servet editorial - Grupo Asís Biomedia, SL
www.grupoasis.com
info@grupoasis.com

GRUPO asis

Servet is the publishing house of Grupo Asís

ACKNOWLEDGEMENTS

We would like to thank all our colleagues at the Clinical Hospital of the Veterinary Faculty in Zaragoza for their continuous support and unselfish collaboration.

Thanks to Dr Manuel Gascón and Dr José Ignacio Bonafonte, both lecturers at the Pathology Department of the Veterinary Faculty in Zaragoza, who encouraged us to venture into the world of radiology.

To Dr Jerry Davies at Davies Veterinary Specialists, for his many hours of patience and dedication.

To all our colleagues at the Medical and Surgical Pathology Units, for their friendship.

To our colleagues in the veterinary profession, who so often have put their trust in us.

And our thanks to the Servet team, for making our project possible in the most professional way.

PREFACE

This book is the result of the authors' work over the recent years in the field of diagnostic imaging, while based at the radiological service of the Veterinary Hospital at the University of Zaragoza.

During these years, we have received a large amount of radiographic material from colleagues in practice who were looking for diagnostic support. On some occasions, the radiographic examination had to be repeated to reach a diagnosis, because an unsuitable technique had been used. "Radiographic technique" covers various aspects, some of which will become much simpler in the near future with the introduction of digital radiography. However, the handling of the patient during a radiographic examination will continue to be of crucial importance, while the technical literature on this subject is extremely limited.

This handbook aims to be a useful tool in daily veterinary practice, by providing clearly outlined information, that can be consulted at a glance, on the most appropriate positions and projections to examine different body structures. Thus the clinician can obtain good quality radiographs for a correct radiological diagnosis.

The book has been divided in six chapters: head, spinal column, thorax, abdomen, forelimb and hind limb, in order to make it easier for the clinician to find the area of interest quickly. In each chapter, the most common projections are described, in combination with the more specific and difficult ones. A series of photographs accompanies the text, one showing the position of the patient lying on the X-ray table and the other the resulting radiograph.

It is our hope that our colleagues will enjoy this handbook and that it will help to simplify radiographic examination that so often provides the definite diagnosis.

Amaia Unzueta Galarza
José Ramón Sever Bermejo

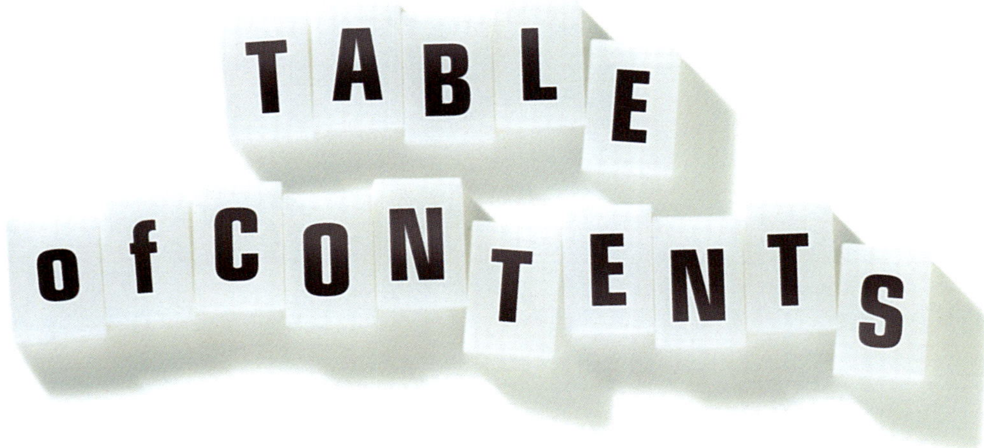

INTRODUCTION

Introduction 2

Preparation of the patient 2

Immobilisation and positioning of the patient 3

Selection of radiographic equipment 5
- X-ray equipment 5
- Scattered radiation, collimators and grids 5
- Cassettes and intensifying screens 6
- Direct exposure film 6

Geometric factors 7

Selection of exposure factors 7

EXAMINATION OF THE HEAD

General considerations 10
- Standard projections: Lat, VD, DV 10

Occipital bone and foramen magnum 13

Tympanic bullae and odontoid process 14

Temporomandibular joint 16

Maxilla 17

Mandible 19

Nasal cavity and sinuses 20

EXAMINATION OF THE THORAX

General considerations 24
- Exposure factors 24
- Positions and projections 25
  - Lateral projection (Lat) 25
  - Dorsoventral projection (DV) 26
  - Ventrodorsal projection (VD) 27

Intrathoracic structures 28
- Trachea 28
  - Oblique dorsocranial-ventrocaudal (skyline) projection 29
- Oesophagus 30
  - Oesophagography 30
- Heart 31
- Lungs 33
- Visualization of the pulmonary blood vessels 34
- Visualization of pleural effusion 34
  - Lateral projection 35
  - Ventrodorsal projection 35

Extrathoracic structures 35

EXAMINATION OF THE ABDOMEN

General considerations 38
Exposure factors 38
Positions and projections 38

Liver and spleen 42

Kidneys and ureters 42
Excretion urography 42

Urinary bladder 44
Retrograde contrast cystography 44

Urethra 46
Contrast urethrography 47

Stomach and small intestine 48
Stomach 48
Small intestine 48
Contrast study of the upper digestive tract 48

Large intestine 52
Colonography 52

Diaphragm 53
Positive peritoneography or celiography 53

EXAMINATION OF THE SPINAL COLUMN

General considerations 56
Exposure factors 56
Positions and projections 56

Cervical column 57

Thoracic column 61

Lumbar column 63

Lumbo-sacral column 66

Myelography 68
Indications 68
Contraindications 68
Technique 68
Cervical myelography 69
Lumbar myelography 70
Complications 71

EXAMINATION OF THE FORELIMB

General considerations 74
Exposure factors 74
Positions and projections 75

Scapula 75

Shoulder 77

Humerus 80

Elbow 82

Radius and ulna 86

Carpus 88

Metacarpus and phalanges 90

EXAMINATION OF THE HIND LIMB

General considerations 94
Exposure factors 94
Positions and projections 94

Pelvis 95

Femur 100

Stifle 102

Tibia and fibula 106

Tarsus 108

Metatarsus and phalanges 111

INTRODUCTION

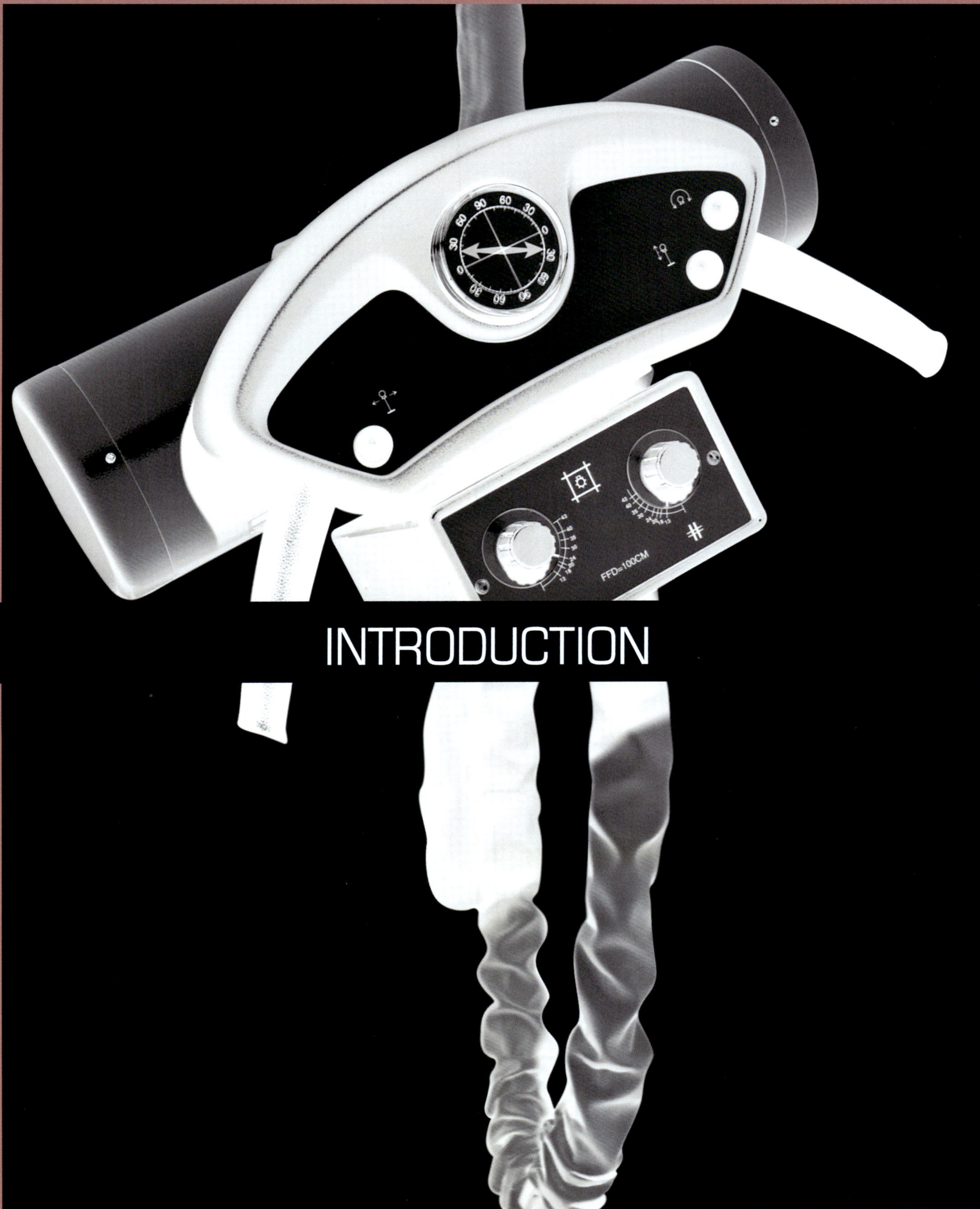

Introduction

There is no doubt that radiographic examination of the dog can be a valuable tool in daily veterinary practice, as it often provides definitive information for the diagnosis of many conditions.

Naturally, radiological interpretation requires many years of study and practice and yet, sometimes it is forgotten that an "excellent radiologist" with an "excellent background" cannot excel if he does not have a good quality radiographic image.

Radiologic quality is defined as a true representation of the patient's anatomical structures on a radiograph, so optimal radiographic quality is essential for a precise diagnosis.

To obtain a good quality radiograph, several factors should be taken into account, such as the characteristics of the patient, the imaging equipment, and technical factors regarding geometry, exposure or processing.

Obviously, some of the technical factors that were considered essential up until now, such as selecting the exposure settings or the key factors of wet processing, will become irrelevant in the near future due to the uptake of digital radiography by the veterinary profession. However, the projections that are obtained during radiographic exposure are still decisive, both for the digital and the analogue image. Hence, the aim of this book is to give an illustrated description of the positions and projections of canine patients during radiographic examination of different anatomical structures.

In this chapter however, we also present a short description of some other quality-related factors mentioned in the rest of the book; although not unimportant, they are not included in the main objectives of this book.

Preparation of the patient

It is often forgotten that it may be important to carry out an initial, thorough external examination of the patient before taking a radiograph. Pets frequently have structures or substances stuck to their coat or skin (vegetable matter, dirt), which may interfere with the radiological image and that should be removed first.

Also, the aids used for immobilising or positioning the patient, as well as dog collars or radiopaque ornaments, should, where possible, be kept from interfering with the image.

Immobilisation and positioning of the patient

The need to sedate or anaesthetise the patient will be determined by its temperament, the clinical condition and the type of projection required. Generally, examination of the head or trauma cases will require chemical immobilisation, as will be explained in the next chapters.

Physical immobilisation and correct positioning of the animal can be achieved by using various aids available on the market, for instance: sand bags, plastic or wooden positioning aids, foam blocks or wedges, plastic or wooden troughs (Fig. 1). However, it is always possible to use simple resources like bandages, or use ingenuity and imagination to produce an equally effective homemade system for restraint of the patient, as long as it is radiolucent if the primary beam is to cross it.

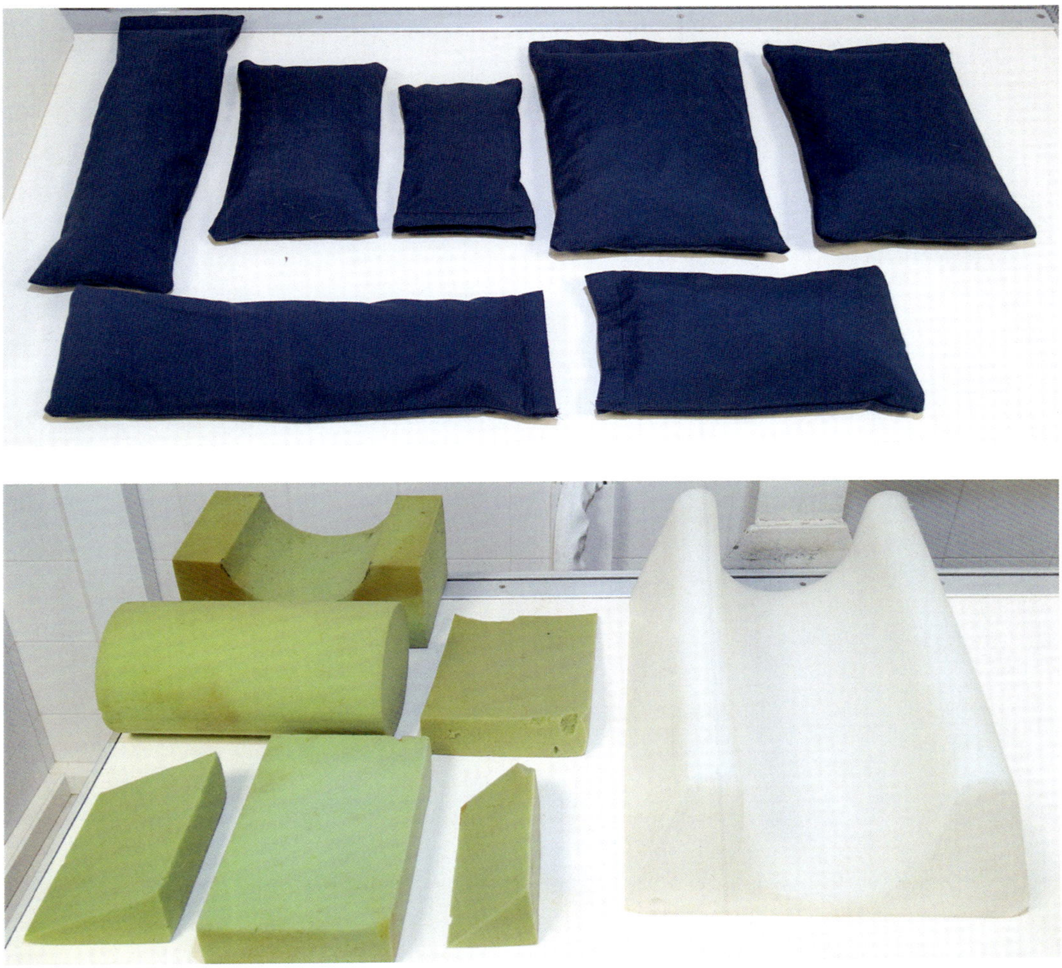

Fig. 1. Sand bags of different sizes, foam wedges of different shapes and a radiolucent positioning aid.

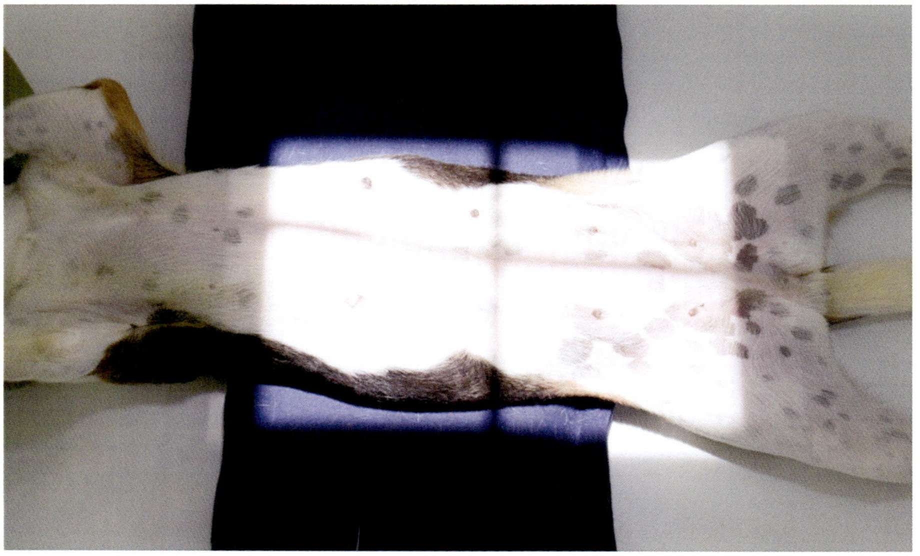

Fig. 2. Ventrodorsal projection of the abdomen. The X-rays enter the abdomen ventrally and exit dorsally.

The position of the patient is determined by the projection that is required. The terminology of radiographic projection refers to the path taken by the X-ray beam through the structure that is being radiographed. The first part of each term describes the surface of the structure where the primary beam enters the tissue, and the second part the surface where it exits. For instance, a ventrodorsal projection of the abdomen indicates that the X-ray beam enters the abdomen ventrally and exits dorsally (Fig. 2).

The term "position" (right or left) used in a lateral projection refers to the side the patient is lying on and not to the projection. For instance, a lateral projection in a right-hand position means that the patient is lying on the table on its right-hand side (Fig. 3).

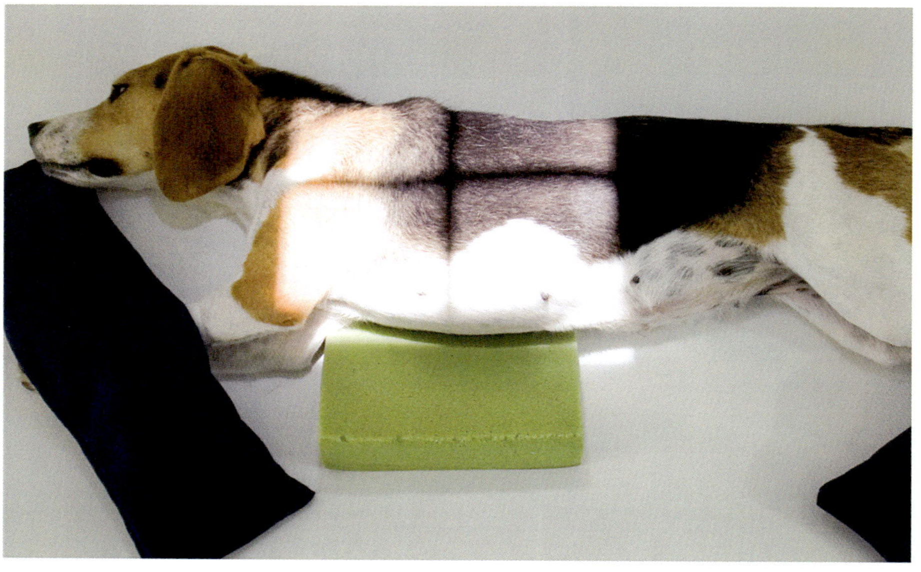

Fig. 3. Lateral projection of the thorax, right-hand position. The patient is lying on its right-hand side.

Selection of radiographic equipment

X-ray equipment

Although it is not the aim of this manual to give a description of an X-ray machine, in the course of the book, various projections that require rotation of the X-ray tube are mentioned. Undoubtedly, certain projections will be easier to do if the X-ray tube can be lowered and pivoted with ease (Fig. 4).

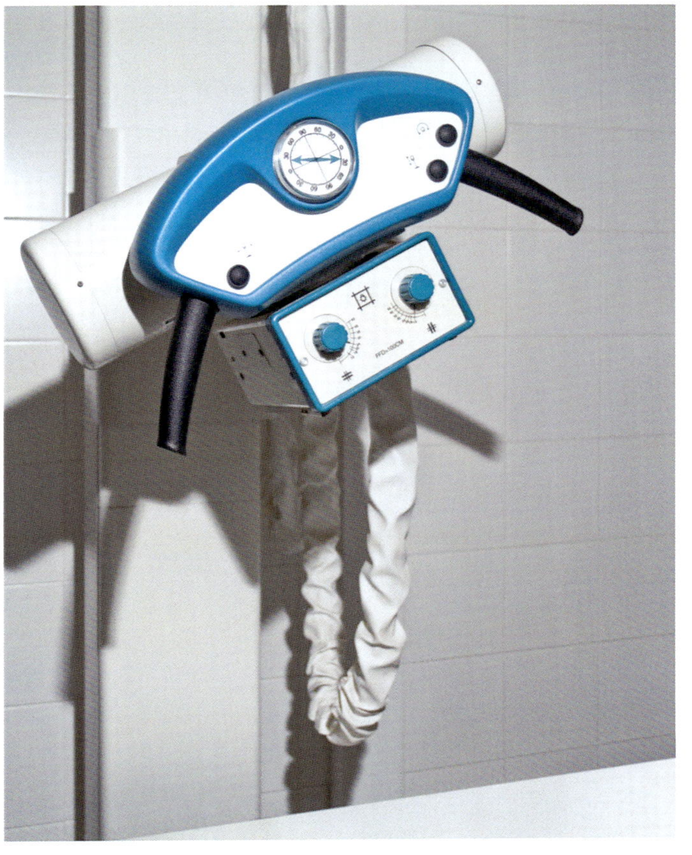

Fig. 4. 30° rotation of the tube.

Scattered radiation, collimators and grids

Scattered radiation is generated by the Compton effect, when X-rays interact with tissue. It causes the appearance of a grey veil on the film, which reduces the contrast and the radiographic quality of the image.

There are two ways to reduce scattered radiation on a radiographic image: the use of a device that restricts the beam and the use of an anti-scatter grid.

Although there are several beam-restricting devices, the one that is most commonly used in veterinary practice and the one that has been used in this handbook, is the variable aperture collimator with a light beam diaphragm that makes it possible to collimate the exposure field both longitudinally and transversally.

The amount of scattered radiation that reaches the film increases with a widening beam, so the beam should be as narrow as possible.

Also, scattered radiation increases with the thickness of the structure being radiographed. Generally, when the thickness is over 10-15 cm, scattered radiation is considered to impair the quality of the image, and the use of an anti-scatter grid is recommended.

A grid is a device made of sections of radiopaque (usually lead) and radiolucent (usually aluminium or plastic) materials. The X-rays that emerge from the patient collide with the radiopaque material in the grid and are absorbed, so that they do not reach the film, while those X-rays that impact with the radiolucent material are transmitted.

Normally, a well-designed grid will reduce scatter by 80-90%. However, it should be remembered that the grid, apart from absorbing the scattered radiation, will also absorb some primary radiation. Therefore, exposure factors should be increased in compensation (the mAs up to 30%), which means that the patient will receive a higher radiation dose.

In this handbook, an in-built grid in the radiography table has been used to radiograph structures thicker than 10 cm. For structures under 10 cm, no grid has been used; the cassette has been placed directly on the tabletop.

Cassettes and intensifying screens

The cassette acts as a protective support for the intensifying screen and the film. The screens are called "intensifying" because they transform the radiation energy they receive from the patient into luminous energy, which interacts with the radiographic film. The use of screens allows a considerable reduction in exposure factors and thus in the radiation dose that the patient and the technical staff (if any) taking the radiograph receive, as well as providing a marked improvement in contrast.

At present, screens are manufactured with a phosphorous material called rare earth, which is why these screens are called rare-earth screens. To put them to the best possible use, they should be used with films that have the corresponding spectral sensitivity. Orthochromatic film (sensitive to blue and green) has an adequate spectral sensitivity for rare-earth screens. In this manual, rare-earth screens have been used in combination with orthochromatic films.

Direct exposure films

Direct exposure films do not have many applications in veterinary practice. They need between 10 and 100 times the radiation dose that used for intensifying screens. The authors use them exclusively for some dental examinations that do not require high exposure factors.

Geometric factors

The two main geometric factors that can alter the quality of a radiograph are: magnification and distortion of the image.

- **Magnification**. All radiographic images are bigger than the object they represent, a phenomenon called magnification.
  In most clinical radiographic examinations, it is advisable that the magnification be kept to a minimum. To achieve this, two basic rules apply: the distance between the source of the radiation and the film, or the film focal distance (FFD) should be large, and the distance between the object to be radiographed and the film, or the film object distance or FOD) should be small.
  When increasing the FFD, the exposure settings have to be increased, too. For this reason, in veterinary practice a FFD of 100-120 cm is used, as this guarantees a reasonable balance between the quality of the image and the exposure settings.

- **Distortion**. The disproportionate increase in size of different parts of the same object is known as distortion. There are two main factors that contribute to this unwanted effect: the thickness and the position of the object.
  Generally, the thicker the object, the bigger the distortion will be. When the thickness is irregular, as happens with many body parts, it is important to centre the X-ray beam on the central part of the structure to minimize distortion.
  Additionally, if the structure and the film are in the same parallel plane, the image will not be distorted, but if they are not parallel, distortion will take place. This is why correct positioning of the patient is essential.

Selection of exposure factors

The size of the patient to be radiographed will determine the settings of the exposure factors. As each X-ray machine has its own radiographic chart, the radiographic settings used by the authors have not been included. However, at the start of each chapter, some comments on exposure factors are included in the general considerations.

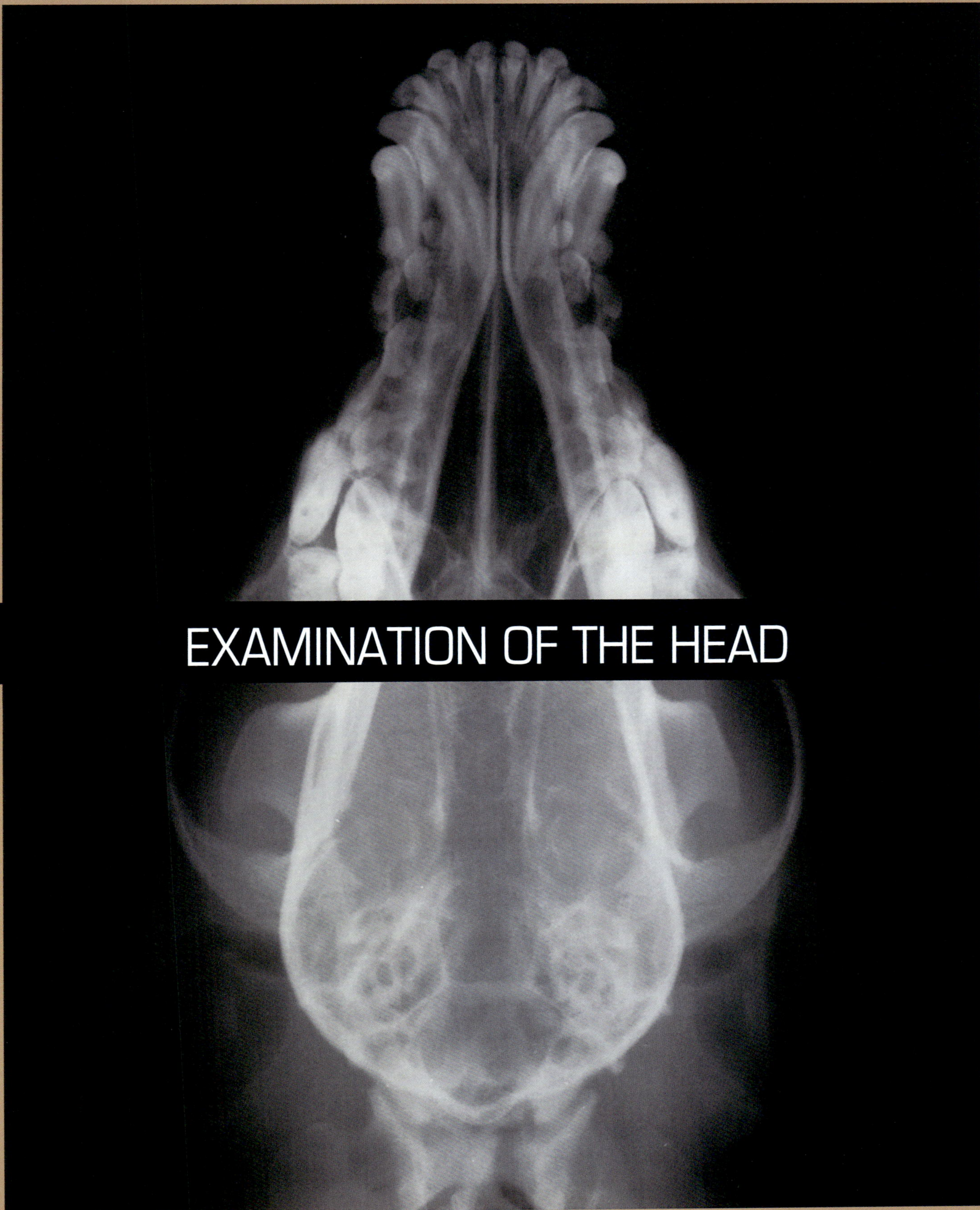

EXAMINATION OF THE HEAD

General considerations

The standard projections Lat, VD and DV are used as a routine, but in most cases, these are not sufficient and special projections are required.

Radiological investigation of the different structures of the head should be carried out with the patient under general anaesthesia to obtain the best possible positioning. The routine projections that are used in all examinations of the head are lateral (Lat), dorsoventral (DV) and/or ventrodorsal (VD). However, there are several intracranial structures that require special projections that will be described in this chapter.

The exposure factors required are modified depending on the location of the structure to be examined, as the thickness of the structure the beam has to pass through may vary considerably.

Generally, an anti-scatter grid is not necessary, except in large breeds, when the thickness of the structure to be radiographed may be greater than 10-15 cm. It should be remembered that the exposure factors must be reduced accordingly when no grid is used.

The chapter starts with a description of the radiological technique used for routine projections of the head: Lat, VD and DV. This is followed by an analysis of the best positions and projections for each different structure of the head.

Standard projections: Lat, VD and DV

Radiological examination of the structures of the head requires general anaesthesia.

As mentioned at the start of this chapter, any of the projections used to examine the head require general anaesthesia.

For the **lateral (Lat) projection** of the head (Figs. 1 and 2):

- Place the patient in lateral recumbency, with the affected side on the table.
- Place the head of the patient on the table in natural extension (or directly on the cassette if no grid is used).
- Ensure the muzzle is perfectly parallel to the table. A foam wedge may be placed under the lower jaw to achieve this.
- Ensure that the ears do not interfere with the image, by moving them out of the way dorsally.
- Centre the X-ray beam on the eyes.

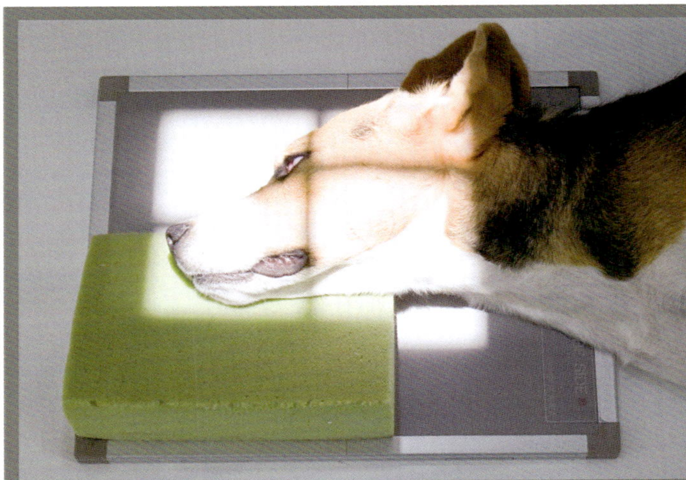

Fig. 1. Patient in lateral recumbency for a lateral projection of the head. The muzzle should be perfectly parallel to the table.

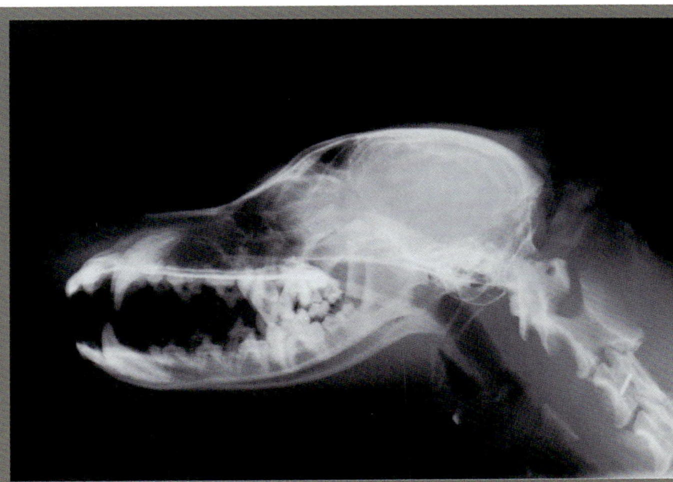

Fig. 2. Radiograph of the Lat projection of the head.

For the **dorsoventral (DV) projection** (Figs. 3 and 4):

- Place the patient in sternal recumbency, using sandbags on both sides of the body to avoid rotation.
- Place the head on the table (or on the cassette if no grid is used).
- Ensure that the head is in a perfectly symmetrical position, avoiding rotation. To achieve this, an imaginary line can be traced between the pupils of the eyes (interpupillary line), which should be perfectly parallel to the surface of the table.
- Ensure that the ears do not interfere with the image by moving them sideways.
- Centre the primary beam on the cranium.

Symmetry of the head can be checked by tracing an interpupillary line, which should be parallel to the surface of the table.

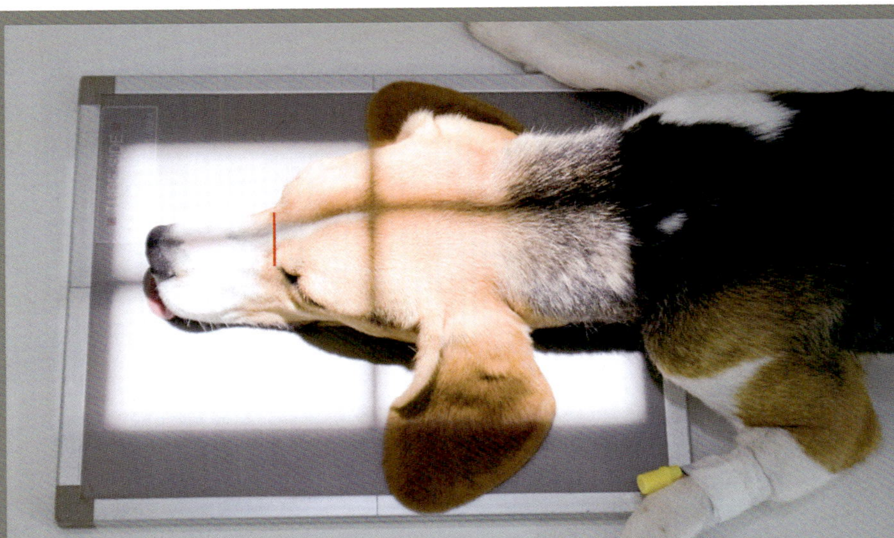

Fig. 3. Animal lying in sternal recumbency for a dorsoventral projection of the head. The imaginary interpupillary line is drawn in red.

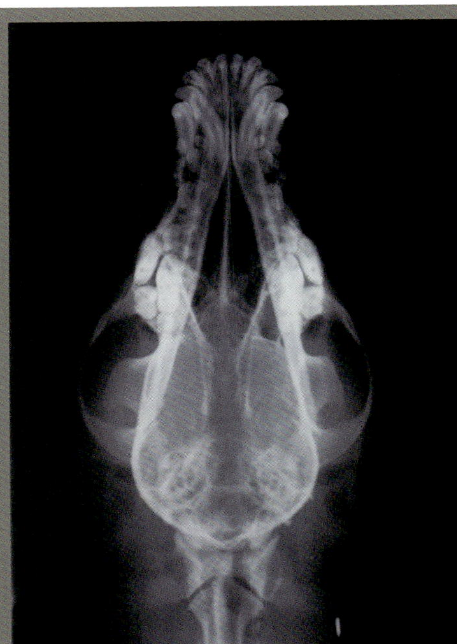

Fig. 4. DV projection of the head.▶

For the **ventrodorsal (VD) projection** (Figs. 5 and 6):

- Place the patient in dorsal recumbency, using sandbags on both sides of the body to avoid rotation.
- Place the head on the table (or directly on the cassette if no grid is used). Press the muzzle down against the table with the aid of a bandage until the jaw is parallel with the tabletop.
- Ensure there is no rotation of the head.
- Check that the ears do not interfere with the image by moving them sideways.
- Centre the primary beam on the intermandibular space.

This is a difficult projection in brachycephalic breeds, for which the dorsoventral projection is recommended.

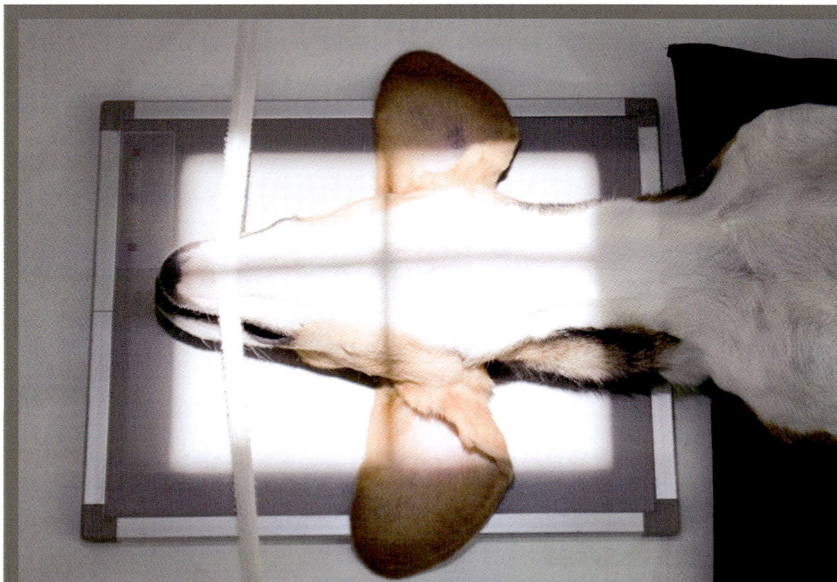

Fig. 5. Animal in dorsal recumbency to achieve a ventrodorsal projection of the head.

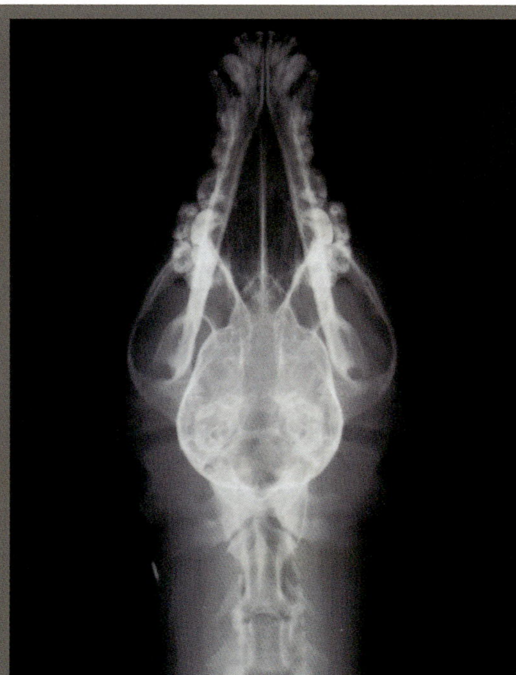

Fig. 6. VD projection of the head. ▶

Occipital bone and foramen magnum

A special **fronto-occipital projection** is needed for the radiological exploration of these two structures.

General anaesthesia is essential to obtain the required position for this projection. Once achieved (Figs. 7 and 8):

- Place the animal in dorsal recumbency with its head on the cassette. Sandbags may be used on both sides of the body to avoid rotation.
- Pull the forelimbs back alongside the body and fix them in this position with whatever means available (sandbags, bandage, rope…).
- Place the muzzle in a vertical position. Then tie a bandage around it and pull it down until the hard palate is at a 30-45° angle to the tabletop.
- Make sure the ears do not interfere with the image by moving them sideways.
- Centre the primary beam on the occipital bone.

The angle between the hard palate and the tabletop should be varied according to the shape of the patient's head.

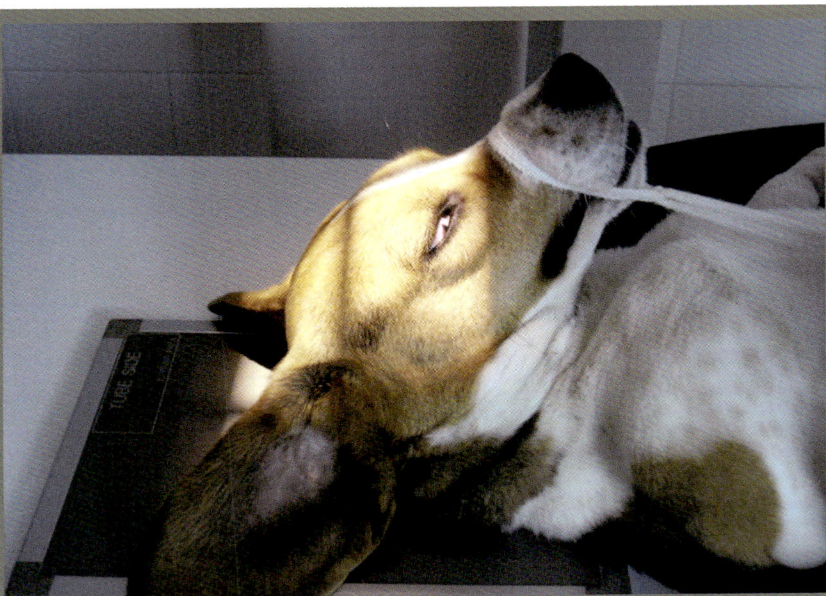

Fig. 7. Position of the head for examination of the occipital bone.

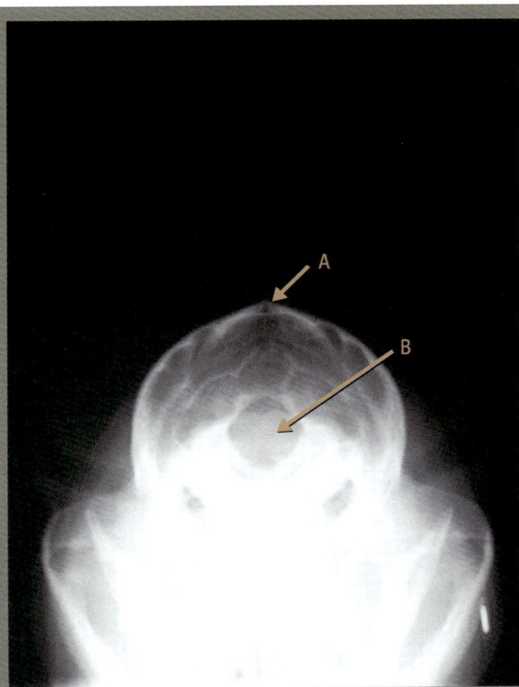

Fig. 8. Fronto-occipital projection. A: occipital bone, B: foramen magnum. ▶

Tympanic bullae and odontoid process

For a complete radiological examination of the tympanic bullae, two special projections are required: an oblique lateral projection and a rostrocaudal open-mouth projection.

Before making a diagnosis, it is advisable to take a radiograph of the contralateral bulla and compare the two.

For the **oblique lateral projection** (Figs. 9 and 10):

- Place the patient in lateral recumbency, with the affected side on the table.
- Place the head on the cassette in such a way that the median plane of the head is in a parallel position to the tabletop, then rotate the dorsal surface of the head some 30° towards the table, so that the affected side moves into a ventral position. A foam wedge can be placed under the lower jaw to maintain the head in position.
- Make sure that the ears do not interfere with the image by moving them out of the way dorsally.
- Centre the primary beam on the area to be explored under the eye.

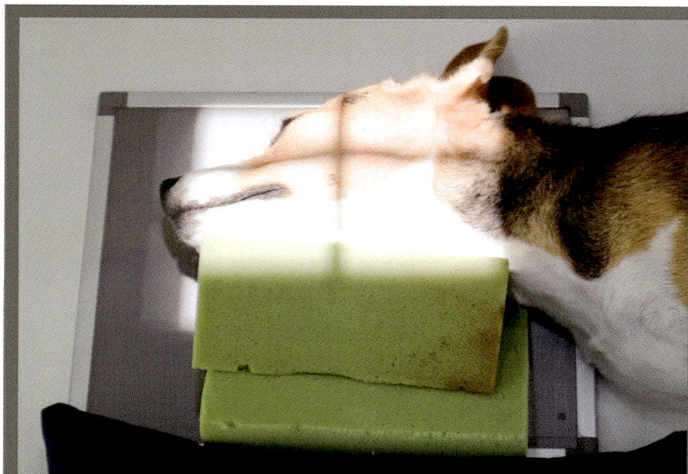

Fig. 9. Positioning of the head for an oblique lateral projection that allows investigation of the tympanic bullae.

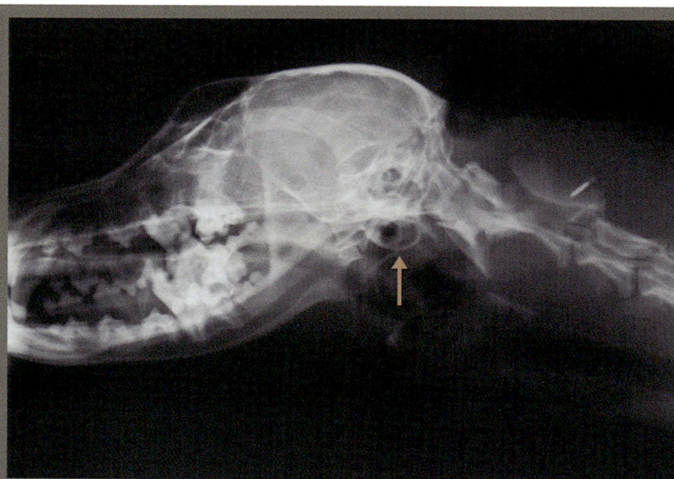

Fig. 10. Oblique Lat projection of the head. The arrow points at the tympanic bulla under study.

The rostrocaudal open-mouth projection is the projection of choice to for visualizing the tympanic bullae, because it avoids overlap with other structures, and because it allows for a comparison between the two bullae on the same radiograph.

At the same time, this projection provides excellent visualization of the odontoid process of the axis.

For the **rostrocaudal open-mouth projection** (Figs. 11 and 12):

- Place the patient in dorsal recumbency with its head on the table. Sandbags may be used on both sides of the body to avoid rotation.
- Pull the forelimbs back alongside the body and fix them in this position with whatever means available (sandbags, bandage, rope…).
- Place the muzzle in a vertical position facing the X-ray tube, in such a way that the hard palate is parallel to the primary beam (in dolichocephalic breeds) and fix it in position with a bandage. In mesocephalic dogs, the angle between the hard palate and the perpendicular beam should be about 10°, while in brachycephalic breeds the angle should be 20°.
- With the aid of another bandage, pull the lower jaw backwards to open the mouth, or pull the tongue backwards, as is shown in Fig. 11.
- Make sure the ears do not interfere with the image by moving them sideways.
- Centre the primary beam on the base of the tongue or the soft palate.

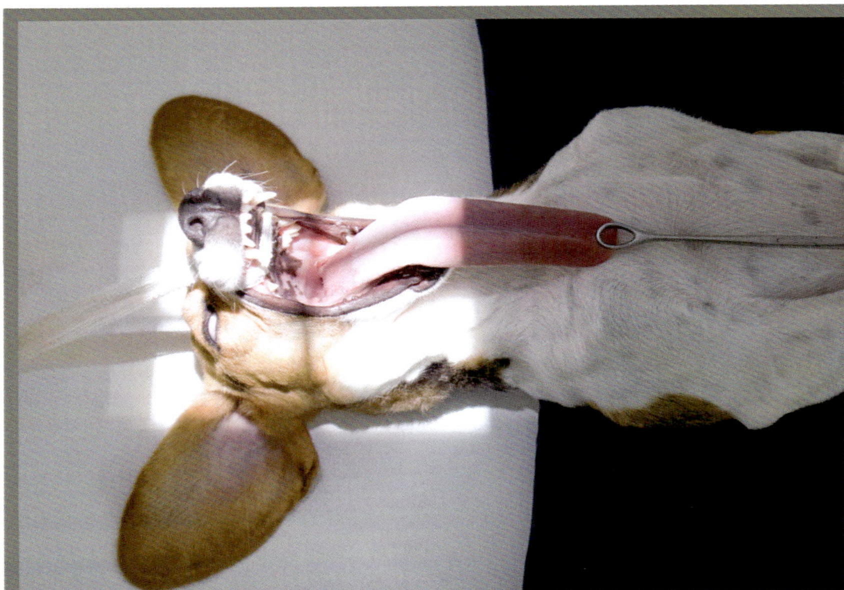

Fig. 11. Positioning of the patient for the rostrocaudal projection.

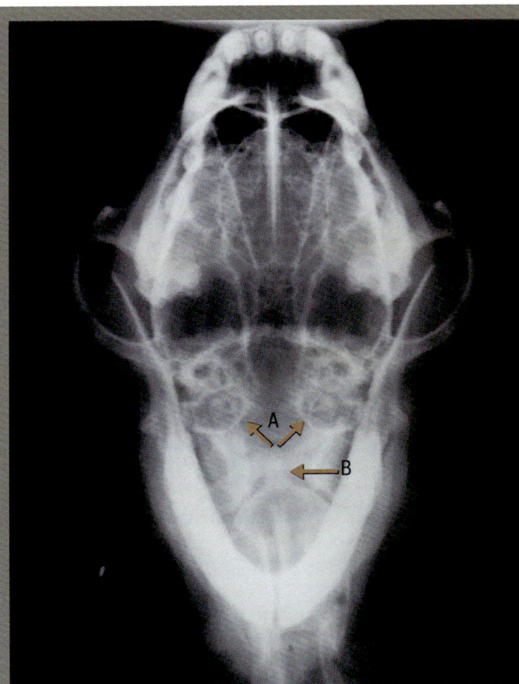

Fig. 12. Rostrocaudal projection of the head for examination of the tympanic bullae (A) and the odontoid process of the axis (B). ▶

The exposure factors used for this projection should be reduced compared to those used for the other projections, as the structure to be X-rayed is much thinner.

Temporomandibular joints

For the radiological examination of the temporomandibular joints, oblique projections are used to avoid superposition of one joint on the other.

The **oblique lateral** projection provides the best visualization of this joint. It is a similar projection to the one described for the tympanic bullae, but with some specific differences (Figs. 13 and 14):

- Place the patient in lateral recumbency, with the affected side on the table.
- Place the head on the cassette with a foam wedge under the muzzle, so that the median plane of the head is tilted up from the table. The degree of tilt (and therefore the size of the foam wedge) depends on the breed: dolichocephalic breeds should be lifted by approx. 10°, mesocephalic breeds some 15° and brachycephalic breeds 25°. The head should then be rotated slightly (approx. 10°) in a dorsal direction, so that the joint to be explored moves into a ventral position. Another foam wedge can be placed under the jaw to maintain the position.
- Ensure that the ears do not interfere with the image by moving them out of the way dorsally.
- Centre the primary beam ventrally to the eye.

This projection can be carried out with the mouth of the patient closed or open. However, an open mouth allows a better visualization of the joint.

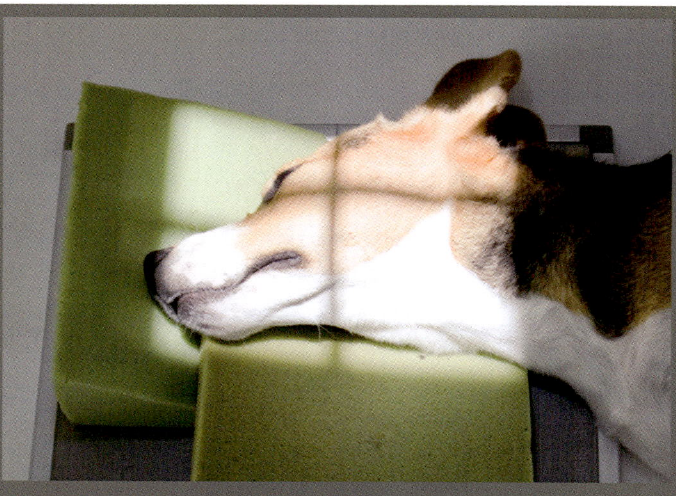

Fig. 13. Oblique lateral projection with a closed mouth to examine the temporomandibular joint.

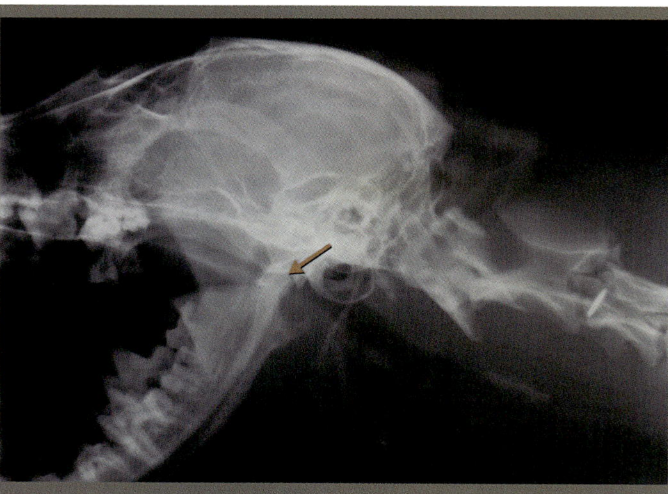

Fig. 14. Oblique Lat projection for investigation of the temporomandibular joint (arrow). The mouth is open.

Maxilla

To examine the maxillary arcades, an oblique lateral and an intraoral dorsoventral projection can be added to the standard Lat and VD/DV projections. It should be kept in mind that in standard Lat and VD/DV projections various structures overlap the maxillary arcade, so that interpretation may be difficult.

For the intraoral dorsoventral projection, the cassette must be inserted in the mouth, which is often impossible due to the small size of the animal or in brachycephalic breeds. This inconvenience can be avoided by the use of dental film.

For the intraoral **dorsoventral projection** (Figs. 15 and 16):

- Place the patient in sternal recumbency, using sandbags on both sides of the body to avoid rotation.
- Place the head on the table and insert the cassette or dental film in the mouth, as far back as possible and parallel to the tabletop. A sandbag on the animal's neck may help to obtain the correct position.
- Ensure the tongue is underneath the cassette or the film to keep it out of the image.
- Take the ears out of the way by moving them sideways, to avoid interference with the radiograph.
- Centre the primary beam on the midline of the dorsum of the nose.

This projection also provides excellent visualization of the upper incisors.

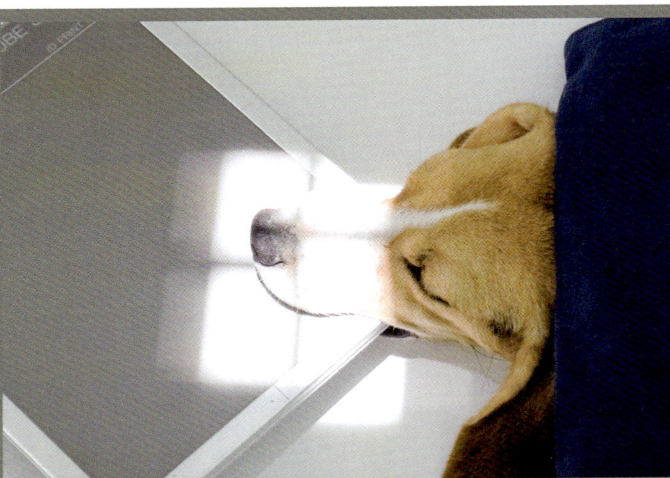

Fig. 15. Position of the patient and the cassette for an intraoral dorsoventral projection.

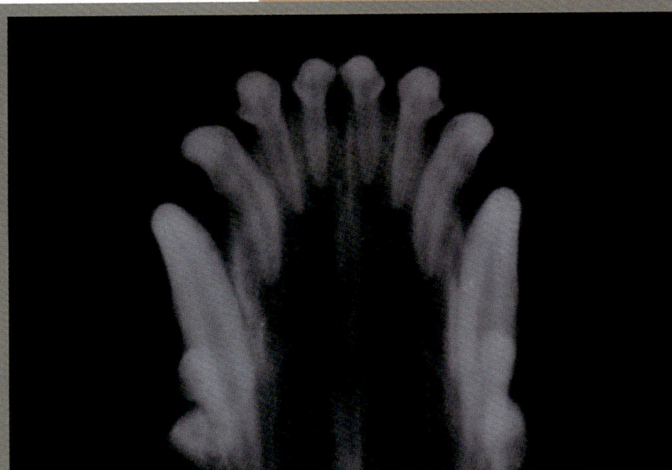

Fig. 16. Intraoral dorsoventral projection.

For the **oblique lateral projection** of the maxilla (Figs. 17 and 18):

- Place the patient in lateral recumbency, with the affected side on the table.
- Tie a bandage around the muzzle and another one around the lower jaw.
- Place the head on the cassette in such a way that the median plane of the head is parallel to the tabletop. Pull on the bandages until the mouth opens sufficiently and the head rotates dorsally by about 45°.
- Do not forget to take the tongue out of the way to avoid superposition on the radiograph.
- Take the ears out of the way by moving them dorsally, to avoid interference with the image.
- Centre the primary beam on the upper premolars.

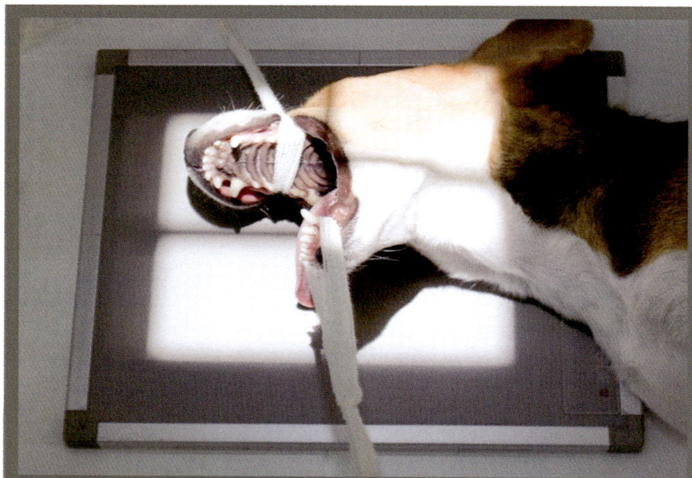

Fig. 17. Position of the head for an oblique lateral projection of the maxilla.

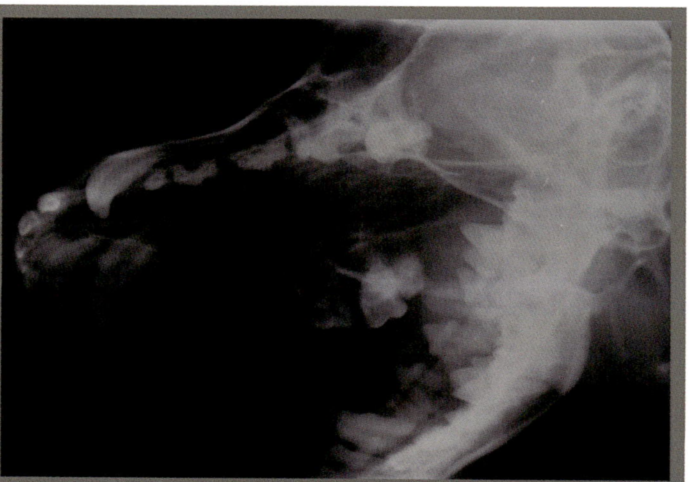

Fig. 18. Oblique Lat projection for examination of the maxilla.

This projection also provides excellent visualization of the upper premolars and molars.

Mandible

To examine the mandibular arcades the standard projections Lat and VD/DV can be used. However, as for the maxilla, these projections suffer from superposition of other structures on the image, which may lead to diagnostic error. Therefore, the oblique lateral and the intraoral ventrodorsal special projections may be added to the standard examination of the mandible.

As with the intraoral DV projection used for the maxilla, the intraoral ventrodorsal projection requires insertion of the cassette in the mouth, which is often impossible due to the small size of the animal or in brachycephalic breeds. This inconvenience can be avoided by the use of dental film.

For the **intraoral ventrodorsal projection** (Figs. 19 and 20):

- Place the patient in dorsal recumbency, using sandbags on both sides of the body to avoid rotation.
- Place the head on the table and insert the cassette or dental film in the mouth, as far back as possible. Pull the muzzle down with the aid of a bandage until the mandible is parallel to the tabletop.
- Ensure that the ears do not interfere with the image by moving them sideways.
- Centre the primary beam on the midline of the intermandibular space.

This projection also provides excellent visualization of the lower incisors.

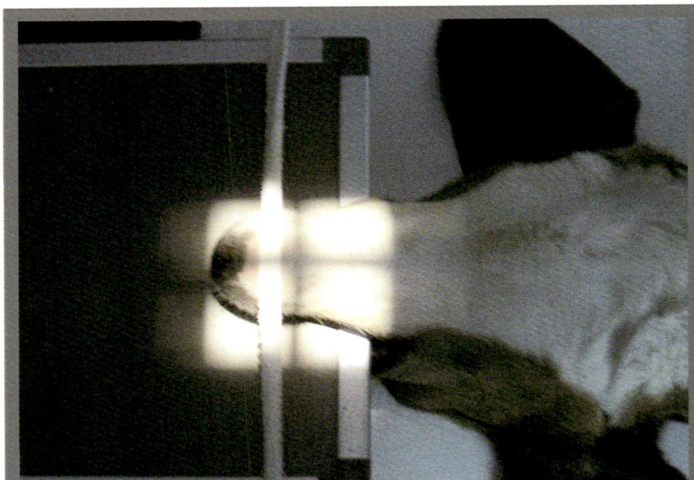

Fig. 19. Position of the patient for an intraoral ventrodorsal projection.

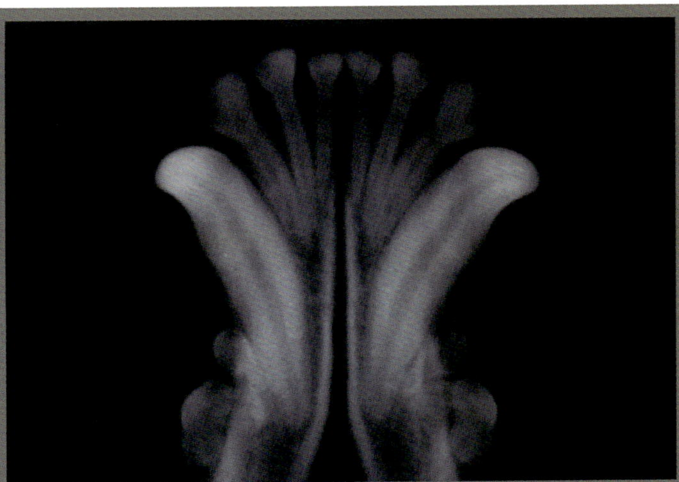

Fig. 20. Intraoral VD projection.

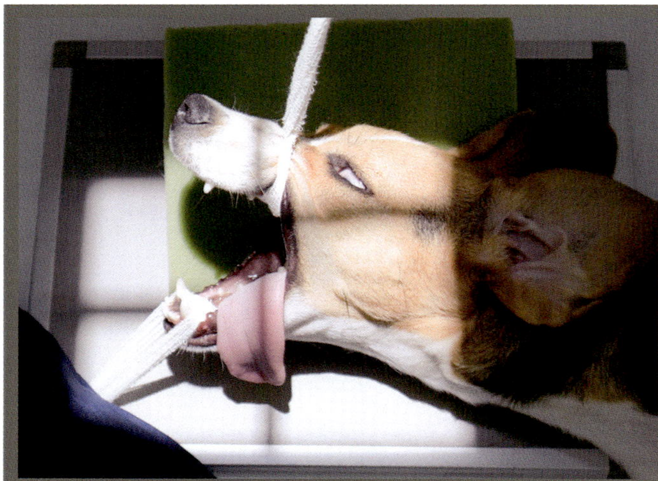

Fig. 21. Position of the head for an oblique lateral projection of the mandible.

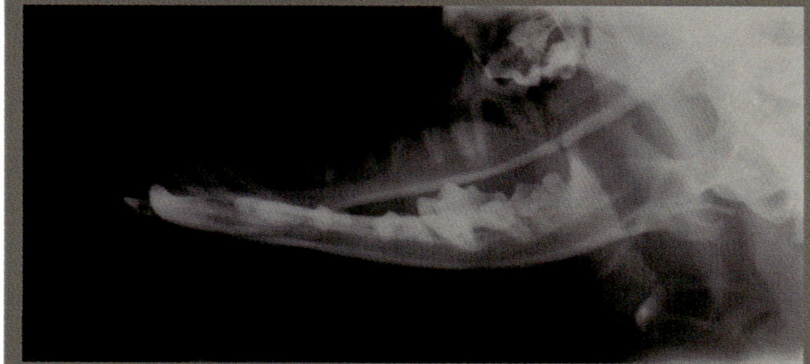

Fig. 22. Oblique Lat projection of the mandible.

For the **oblique lateral projection** of the mandible (Figs. 21 and 22):

- Place the patient in lateral recumbency, with the affected side on the table.
- Place the head on the cassette. Open the mouth and rotate the head by approx. 30-45° in relation to the tabletop, depending on the breed. A foam wedge can be used to keep the head in position.
- Ensure the ears do not interfere with the X-ray by moving them dorsally.
- Centre the primary beam on the lower premolars.

This projection also provides excellent visualization of the premolars and molars of the mandible.

Nasal cavities and sinuses

Radiological examination of the nasal cavities and the sinuses starts with the standard Lat and VD/DV projections for the head. However, these studies should be supplemented by other projections that avoid superposition of other structures. The complementary projections of choice are the intraoral dorsoventral projection described for the maxilla and the rostrocaudal and the open-mouth ventrodorsal projections.

The **intraoral dorsoventral projection** described for exploration of the maxilla (Fig. 15) is also suitable for visualization of the nasal area. The only additional comment would be that, if one wishes to examine the most caudal part of the nasal area, the X-ray tube could be tilted in a rostrocaudal direction at an angle of 10-15°.

For the **open-mouth ventrodorsal projection** (Figs. 23 and 24):

- Place the patient in dorsal recumbency, using sandbags on both sides of the body to avoid rotation.
- Pull the forelimbs back alongside the body and fix them in this position with whatever means available (sandbags, bandage, rope…).
- Place the head on the cassette. With the aid of a bandage behind the upper canine teeth, pull until the hard palate is parallel to the tabletop.
- Tie another bandage behind the lower incisors and pull until the mouth opens sufficiently.
- Tilt the X-ray beam in a rostrocaudal direction by between 20 and 30º in relation to the tabletop, depending on the breed.
- Ensure that the ears do not interfere with the image by moving them sideways.
- Centre the primary beam on the hard palate.

Remember to reduce the exposure factors, as the thickness of the structure to be radiographed is also reduced.

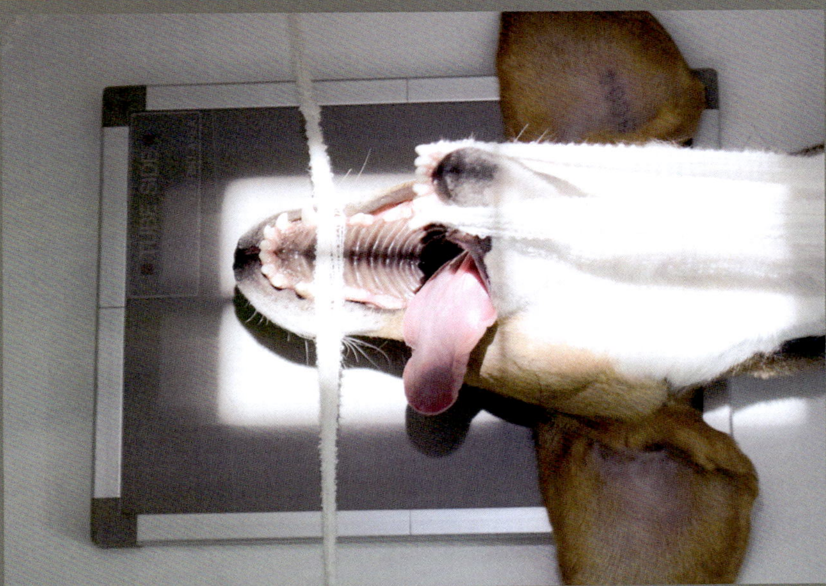

Fig. 23. Position of the head for the open-mouth ventrodorsal projection used for the examination of the nasal cavities and the sinuses.

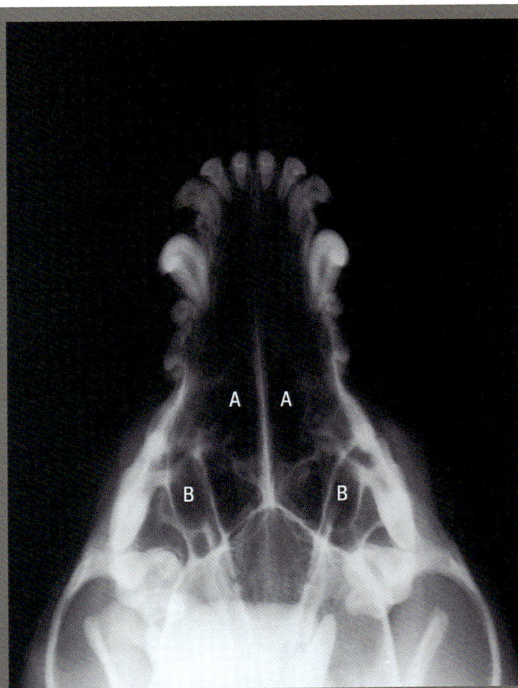

Fig. 24. Open mouth VD projection for the examination of the nasal cavities (A) and the frontal sinuses (B). ▶

For the **frontal rostrocaudal projection** (Figs. 25 and 26):

- Place the patient in dorsal recumbency, using sandbags on both sides of the body to avoid rotation.
- Pull the forelimbs back alongside the body and fix them in this position with whatever means available (sandbags, bandage, rope…).
- Place the head on the cassette and orient the muzzle towards the X-ray tube. With the aid of a bandage tied around the muzzle, pull it down until the hard palate makes an angle of about 20° in relation to the primary perpendicular beam.
- Ensure that the ears do not interfere with the X-ray by moving them sideways.
- Centre the primary beam between the frontal sinuses.
- Reduce the exposure factors accordingly.

This is the best projection for visualization of the frontal sinuses.

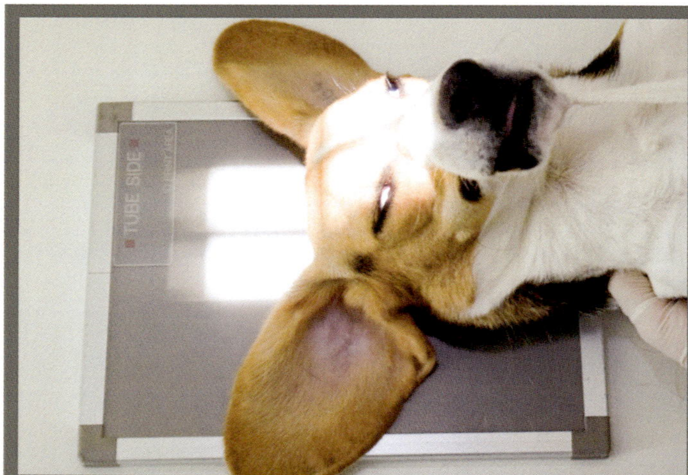

Fig. 25. Position of the patient for frontal rostrocaudal projection.

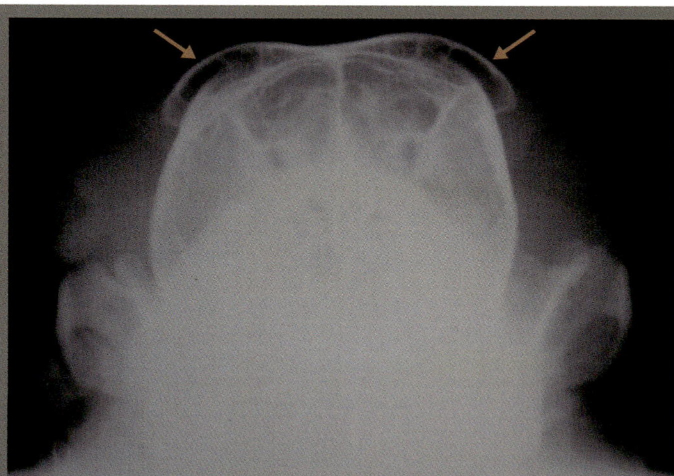

Fig. 26. Frontal rostrocaudal projection for examination of the frontal sinuses.

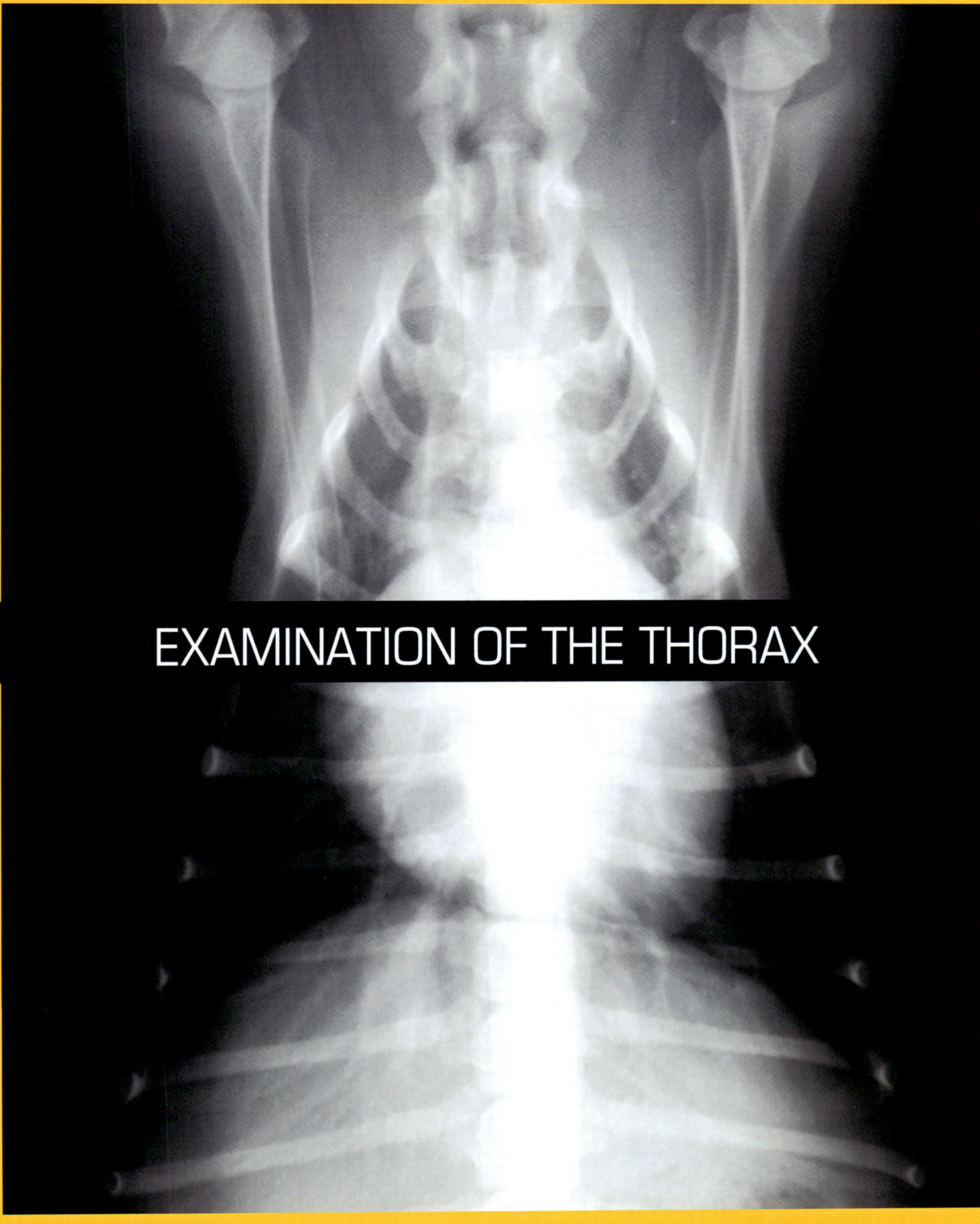

EXAMINATION OF THE THORAX

General considerations

Exposure factors

The negative effect of the patient's respiratory movement on the image can be minimized by using the shortest possible exposure time.

In routine examination of the thorax a **high kilovoltage (kV)** and a **low milliamperage-second (mAs)** should be used. This has two reasons. On the one hand, by using a high kilovoltage, the scale of contrast can be increased to a maximum. On the other hand, whenever the thorax is radiographed, allowances should be made for the loss of detail on the image caused by the inevitable movement of the thorax when the patient breathes in and out (Fig. 1). The use of a low milliampere-second value makes it possible to reduce exposure time to a minimum.

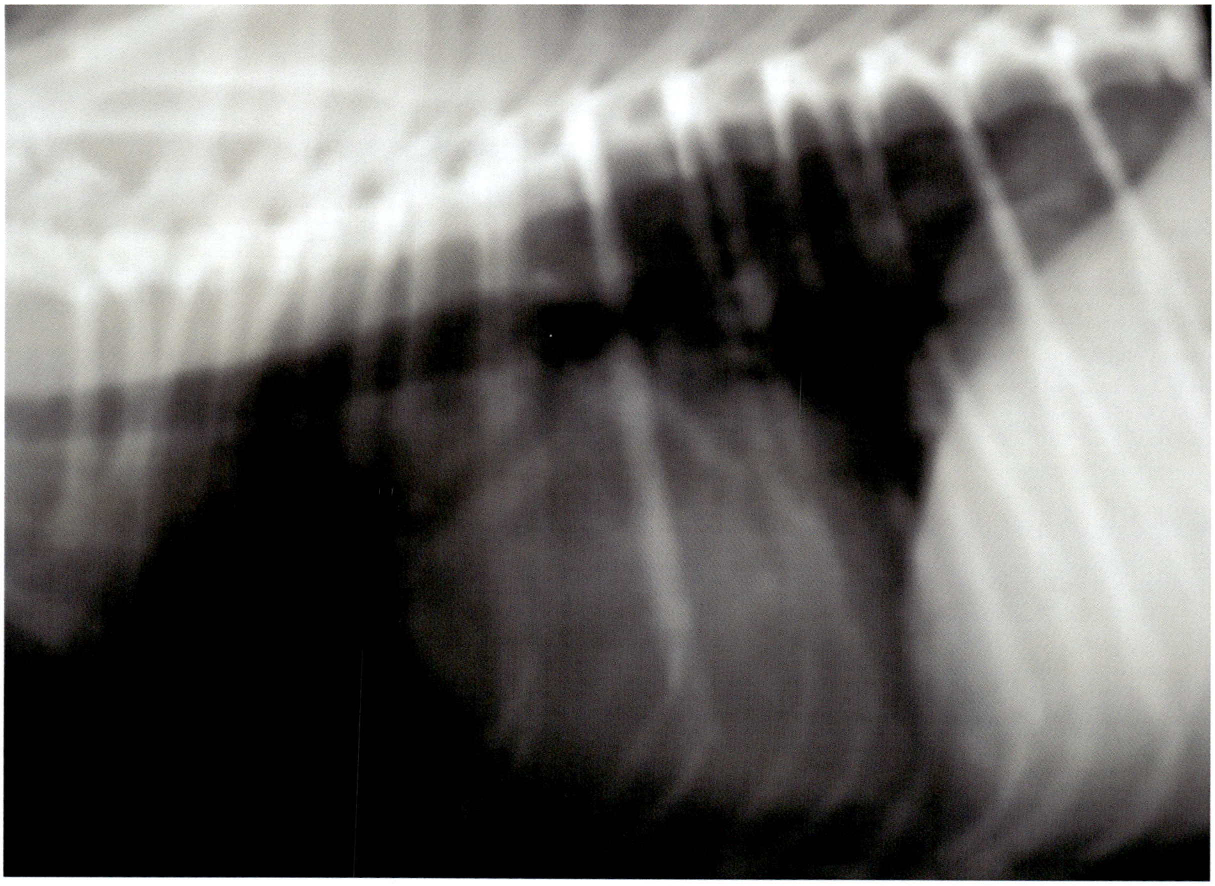

Fig. 1. Loss of detail and sharpness of the structures in the thorax caused by the patient's movement during exposure.

Furthermore, the right choice of exposure factors is essential for a correct interpretation of the thorax. An overexposed image may lead to under-diagnosis, as the visualization of radiopaque lung lesions is impeded (Fig. 2), whereas an underexposed image may lead to over-diagnosis because of an artefactual increase in the radiopacity of the lung (Fig. 3).

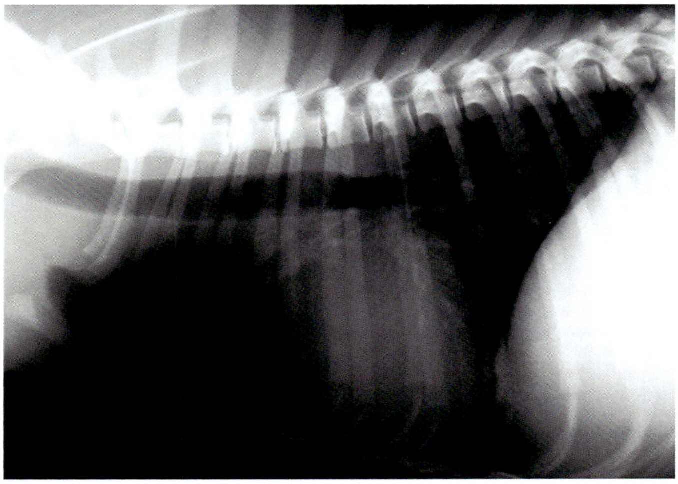

Fig. 2. Loss of radiopacity of the soft tissue can be observed due to overexposure of the film.

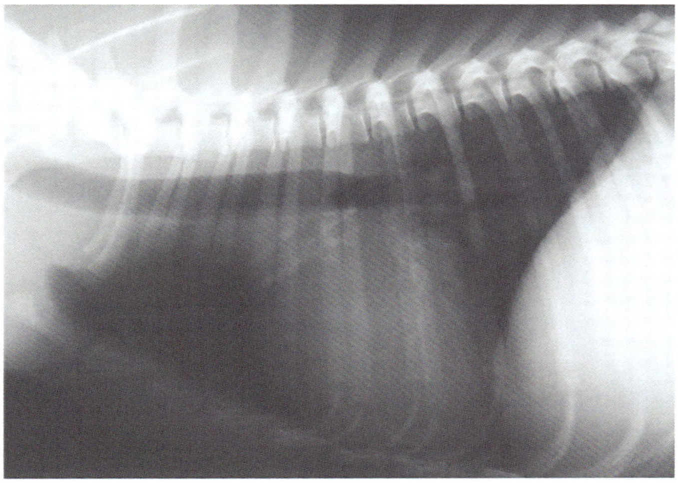

Fig. 3. Underexposure leads to an artefactual increase in thoracic radiopacity.

Positions and projections

Routine radiological examination of the thorax requires at least two perpendicular radiographs.

One of the projections must be lateral (Lat). This projection may be carried out with the patient lying either on its right or on its left side. It should be remembered that, when referring to an X-ray as right or left lateral, the term right or left describes the side the patient is lying on, and not the projection.

The choice of side is of interest, as it may lead to significant differences in the radiological conformation of some intrathoracic structures, which will be discussed further in this chapter.

The radiological projection refers to the place where the X-ray beam enters and exits the patient.

The terms right and left do not refer to the projection, but to the position of the patient on the X-ray table.

Lateral projection (Lat)

For the lateral (Lat) projection of the thorax (Figs. 4 and 5):

- Place the patient on the side of choice, with its spinal column parallel to the tabletop.

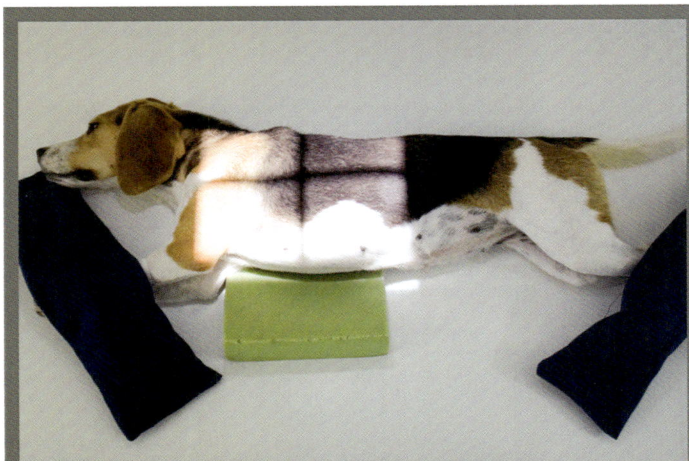

Fig. 4. Patient in lateral recumbency for a Lat projection of the thorax.

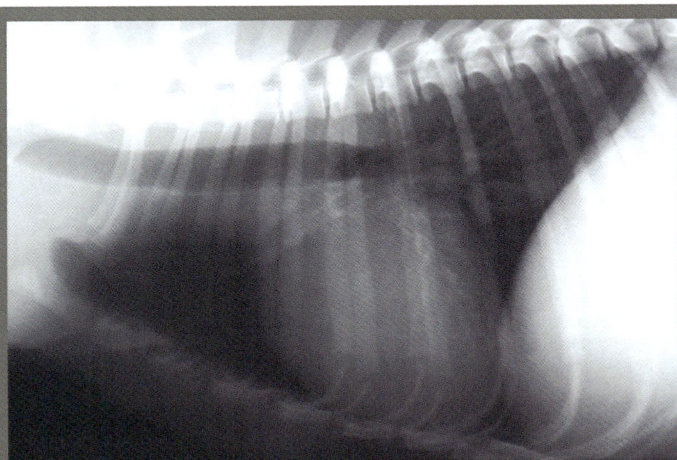

Fig. 5. Lat projection of the thorax.

Radiographs of the thorax should be made at full inspiration.

- Keep the head in a normal position.
- Pull the forelimbs forward to avoid soft tissue superimposition on the cranial thorax, which will lead to artefactual soft tissue radiopacity (Figs. 6 and 7).
- Centre the primary beam at the level of the cardiac silhouette (fifth intercostal space). The place where the cardiac apex can be felt beating against the thoracic wall may be of help when centring the beam.
- The complete thorax should be included (from the thoracic inlet to the most caudal part of the caudodorsal lung field).
- Wait for full inspiration to expose the film. A good radiograph of the thorax must coincide with an inspiration of the patient to obtain maximum pulmonary contrast.

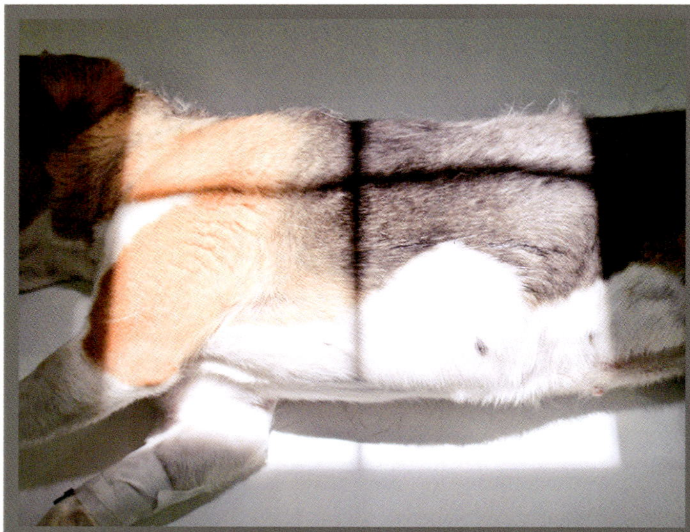

Fig. 6. The leg on the table has moved backwards.

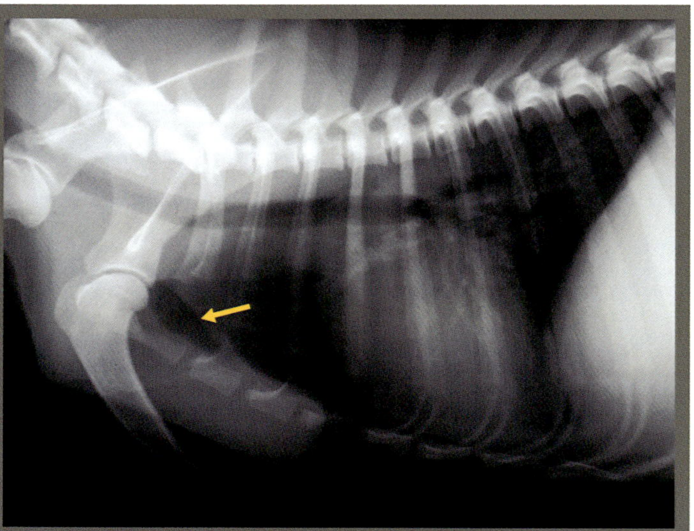

Fig. 7. The increased radiopacity that can be seen in the cranial thorax (arrow) is an artefact, caused by the soft tissue of the foreleg that has moved backwards.

After the Lat projection, a perpendicular view should be obtained: either a dorsoventral (DV) or a ventrodorsal (VD) projection.

Dorsoventral projection (DV)

For the dorsoventral (DV) projection (Figs. 8 and 9):

- Place the patient in sternal recumbency.
- Keep the head on the table in a natural position.
- Pull the forelimbs forward and the hind limbs backwards.
- Centre the primary beam on the cardiac silhouette (5th intercostal space).
- Include the complete thorax.
- Expose the film at the moment of full inspiration.

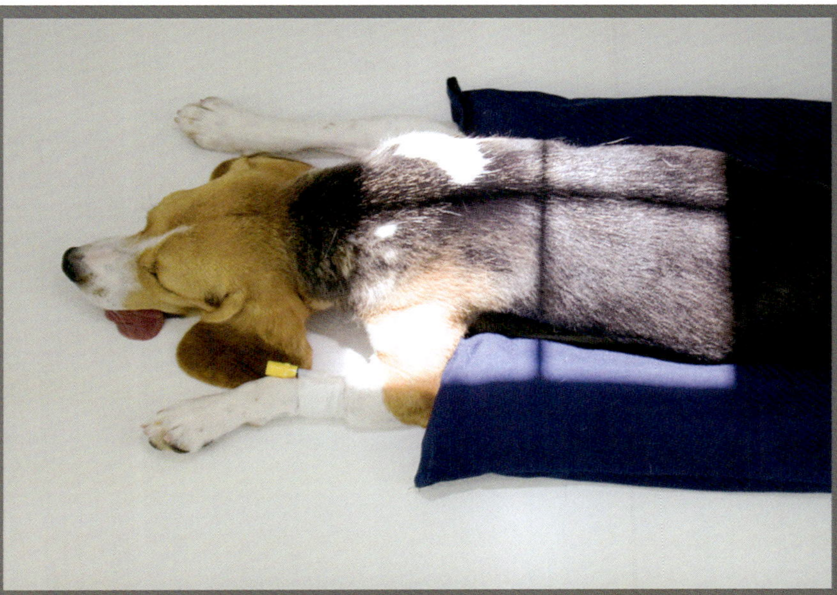

Fig. 8. Animal in sternal recumbency for a DV projection.

Fig. 9. DV projection of the thorax. ▶

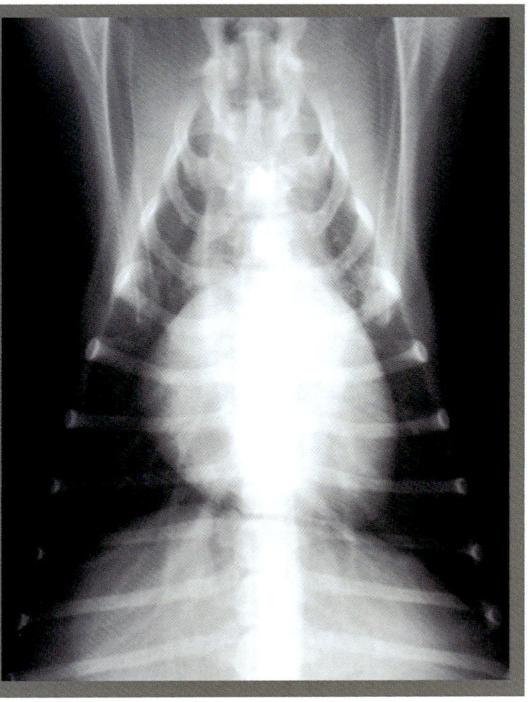

Ventrodorsal (VD) projection

For the ventrodorsal (VD) projection (Figs. 10 and 11):

- Place the patient in dorsal recumbency.
- Keep the head in a natural position.
- Pull the forelimbs forward and the hind limbs backwards.
- Centre the primary beam on the xyphisternum.
- Include the complete thorax.
- Expose the film at the moment of full inspiration.

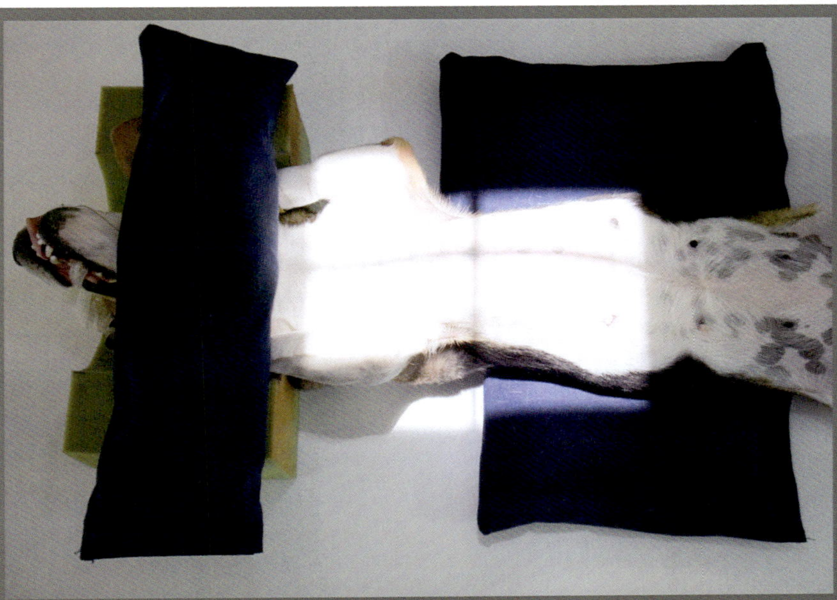

Fig. 10. Animal in dorsal recumbency for a VD projection.

Fig. 11. VD projection of the thorax. ▶

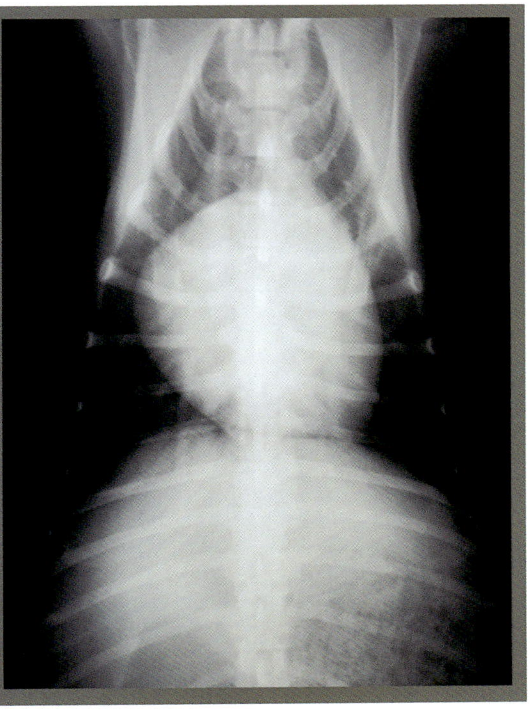

Intrathoracic structures

Trachea

For a correct interpretation of the intrathoracic trachea, forced extension or flexion of the neck should be avoided.

Routine examination of the intrathoracic trachea requires a **Lat projection**. During the procedure, the patient's head and neck should be straight, avoiding either flexion or over-extension. Forced extension of the neck may cause a false image of tracheal constriction and compression at the thoracic inlet (Fig. 12), whereas flexing it may curve the trachea in a dorsal direction, suggesting displacement (Fig. 13).

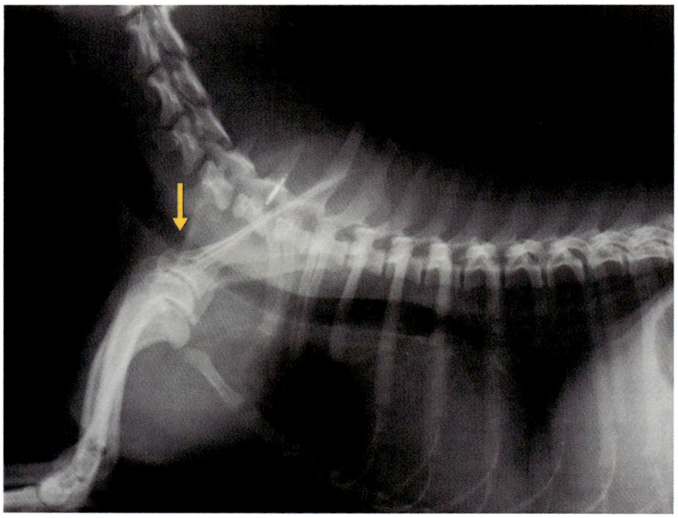

Fig. 12. The artefactual constriction of the trachea is caused by forced extension of the neck.

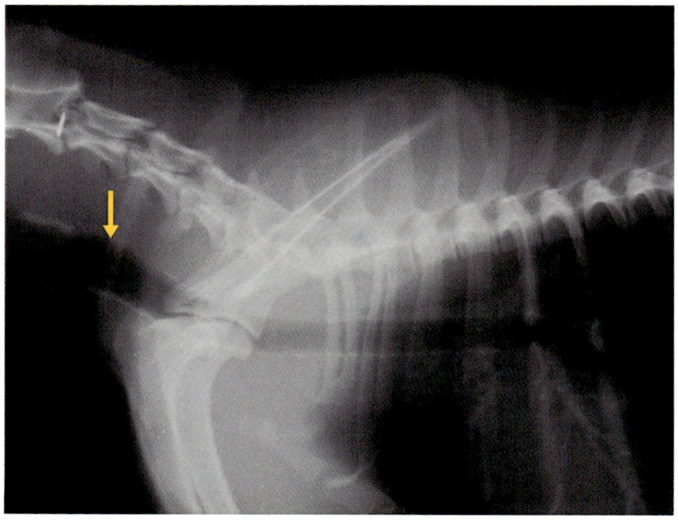

Fig. 13. The trachea curves in a dorsal direction because of forced flexion of the neck.

A VD projection of the thorax is usually not helpful in tracheal examination because, due to its position in the midline, there is superimposition of the spinal column, which hampers its visualization. Still, this projection may be interesting when there is suspicion of a peritracheal compressive mass that causes displacement of the trachea away from the midline. It should be remembered that, in the cranial mediastinum, the trachea may appear slightly deviated towards the right in brachycephalic breeds or obese animals.

Most tracheal problems are dynamic by nature and will produce variations in the tracheal size associated with the respiratory cycle, the so-called **tracheal collapse**. Dynamic narrowing of the tracheal lumen, due to tracheal instability, appears at the thoracic inlet during inhalation and in the area of the carina tracheae during exhalation. This is why lateral radiographs both during inhalation and exhalation are required for a radiological evaluation of tracheal collapse. Apart from the lateral projections, an oblique dorsocranial-ventrocaudal (skyline) projection may be used.

Oblique dorsocranial-ventrocaudal (skyline) projection.

For this projection (Figs. 14 and 15):

- Place the cassette on the table (without a grid). As a grid is not used, remember to reduce the exposure factors (by 15%) with respect to the usual ones!
- Place the patient in ventral recumbency.
- Pull the forelimbs forward and the hind limbs backwards (or flex them in a "frog" position).
- Hyperextend the head.
- Tilt the X-ray tube in a dorsocranial-ventrocaudal direction by about 30 degrees.
- Centre the primary beam on the thoracic inlet.
- Take radiographs both at inhalation and exhalation.

Radiological evaluation of tracheal collapse requires radiographs both at inhalation and exhalation.

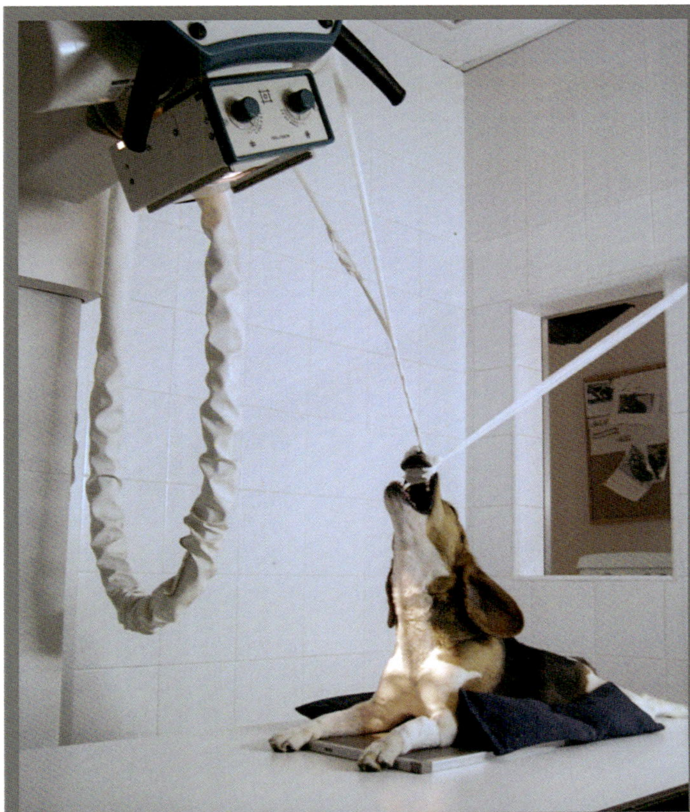

Fig. 14. Position of the patient for a tangential view of the trachea at the thoracic inlet.

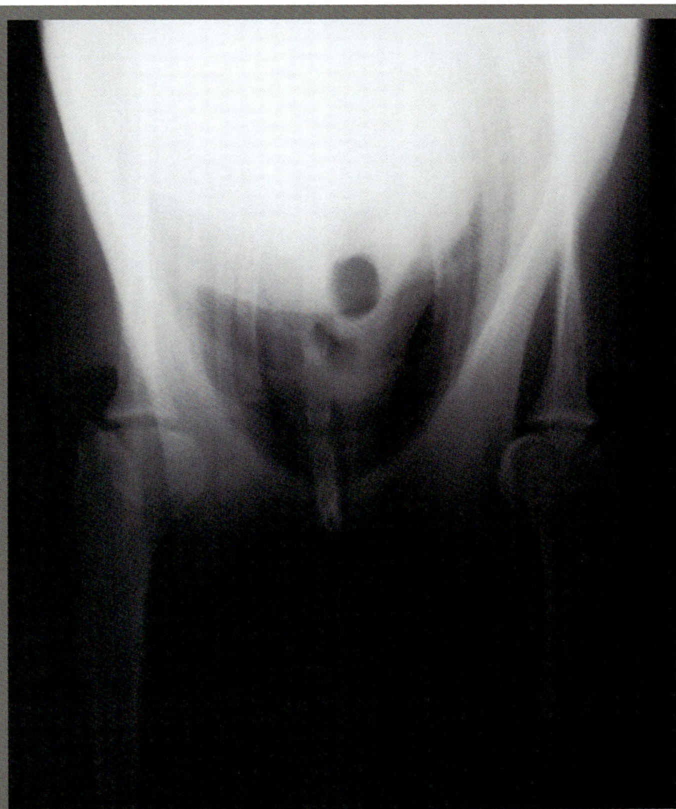

Fig. 15. Radiograph obtained with the skyline projection.

When a perforation of the digestive tract is suspected, barium administration should be avoided. It should be replaced by an iodinated contrast agent.

Oesophagus

Routine radiological examination of the thoracic oesophagus requires a standard lateral projection of the thorax. DV and VD projections do not provide much information, because of the superimposition of the spinal column on the oesophageal shadow; this is why, at times, oblique projections are recommended, as they orient the oesophagus in a visible position.

When basic radiology suggests oesophageal disease, it may be necessary to carry out oesophagography. This technique consists of the oral administration of a positive contrast medium. Motility problems of the oesophagus should be evaluated in the first place with liquid barium, followed by the administration of barium-covered food. When administering the liquid barium, utmost care should be taken to avoid contrast medium entering the airway, which could lead to aspiration pneumonia.

Water-soluble iodinated solutions are indicated when oesophageal perforation is suspected, as they are not very irritant for the body cavities; however, they are not used routinely, because they do not adhere well to mucous membranes.

Oesophagography

For oesophagography:

- Cover the animal with paper or cloth to prevent positive contrast medium staining the coat and causing a radiological artefact (Figs. 16 and 17).

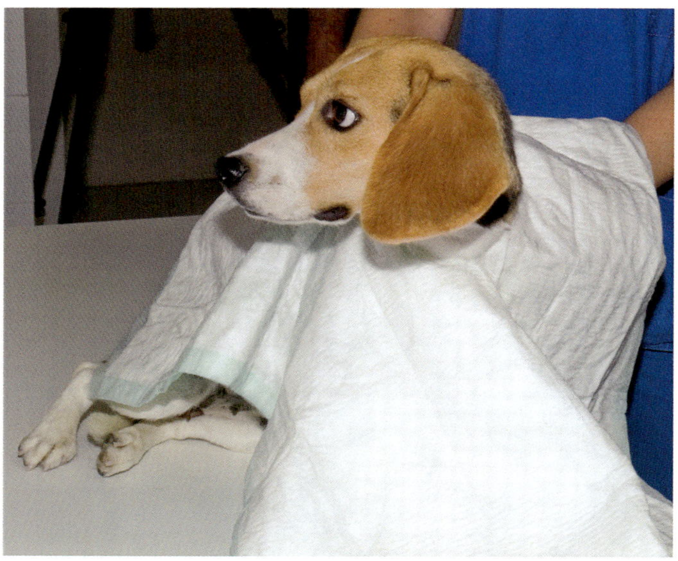

Fig. 16. Before oral administration of the positive contrast medium, the animal's coat should be covered by a bib (photo).

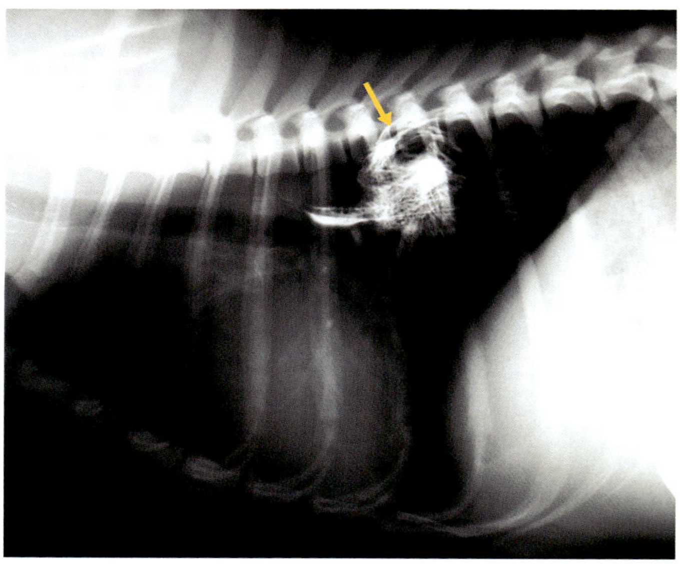

Fig. 17. The presence of positive contrast medium on the animal's coat has been registered on the radiograph and may lead to diagnostic error.

- Administer a liquid suspension of the positive contrast medium (5-20 ml) orally, using a syringe (in the case of a barium medium, administer slowly to avoid inhalation); alternatively, mix a small quantity of tinned food with the contrast medium and let the animal eat it.

Before administration of the positive contrast medium, the patient should be covered with a bib to avoid artefacts on the image.

- Immediately after administration of contrast medium (zero time), take a radiograph in Lat projection, which will show the presence of the medium in the gastric area in the absence of oesophageal abnormalities (Fig. 18).

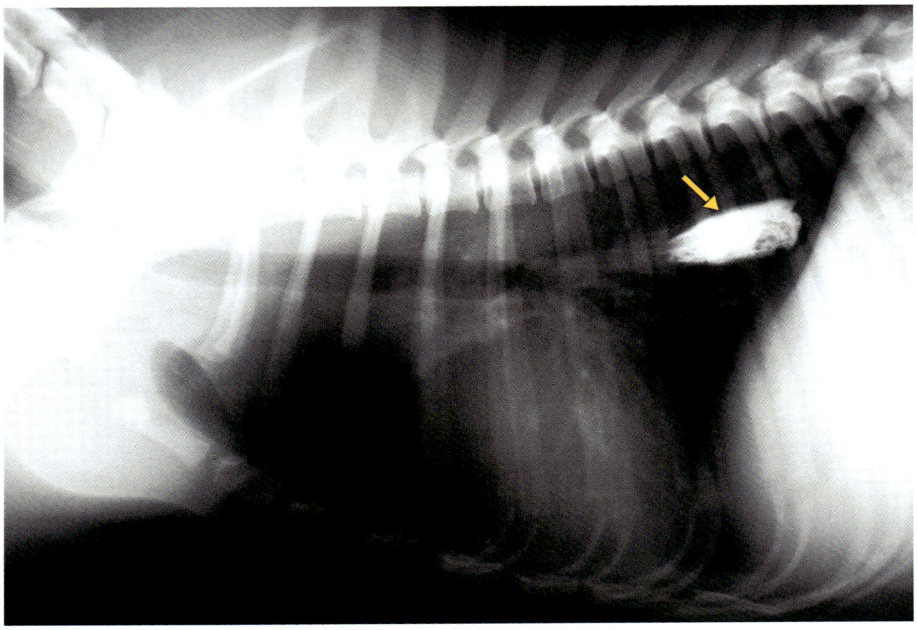

Fig. 18. Presence of a small quantity of positive contrast medium in the oesophagus during an oesophagography at zero time.

Heart

Radiological examination of the heart requires two perpendicular projections. One should be the **standard lateral** projection of the thorax that has already been described.

The perpendicular projection of choice to examine the cardiac silhouette is the **standard DV** projection as opposed to the VD projection, because sternal recumbency used for the DV projection situates the heart closer to the radiographic film, providing an image of the heart size that is close to reality. Sometimes, the VD projection is a better option than the DV, because the dorsal recumbency used for this projection is better tolerated by some patients than sternal recumbency.

With VD projections, it should be remembered that the radiological image of the cardiac silhouette will appear magnified, because the distance between the heart and the radiographic film is larger than in a DV projection.

On the next two pages, some comments on the technicalities to be considered for the diagnostic interpretation of the shape and size of the heart.

The ventrodorsal projection magnifies the cardiac silhouette.

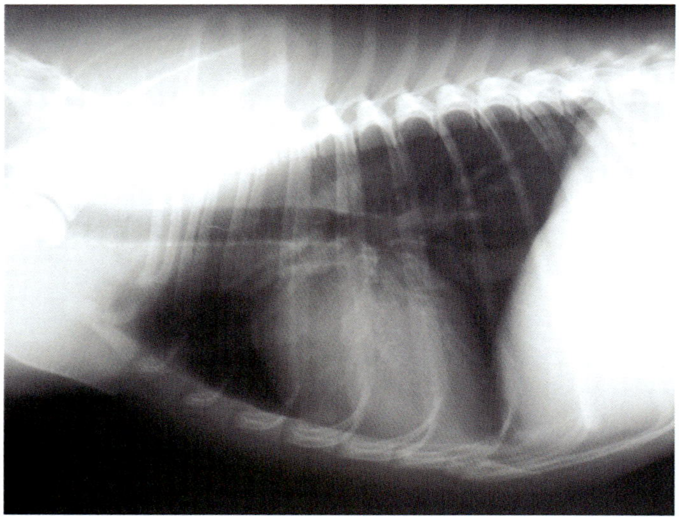

Fig. 19. Right lateral radiograph of the thorax. The cardiac silhouette is egg-shaped.

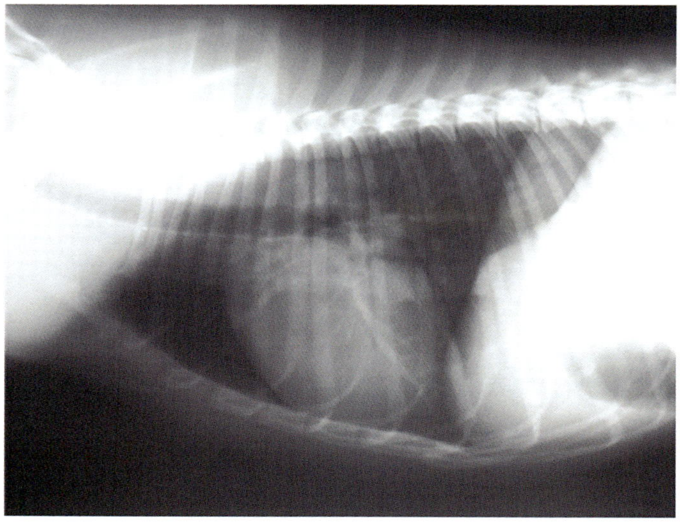

Fig. 20. Left lateral radiograph of the thorax. The cardiac silhouette is rounder.

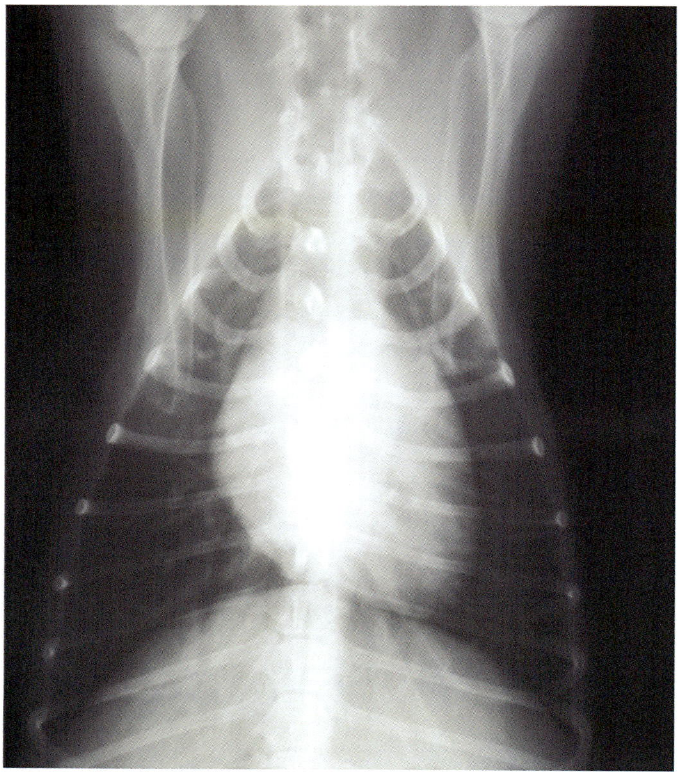

Fig. 21. Dorsoventral projection of the thorax. The cardiac silhouette is egg-shaped.

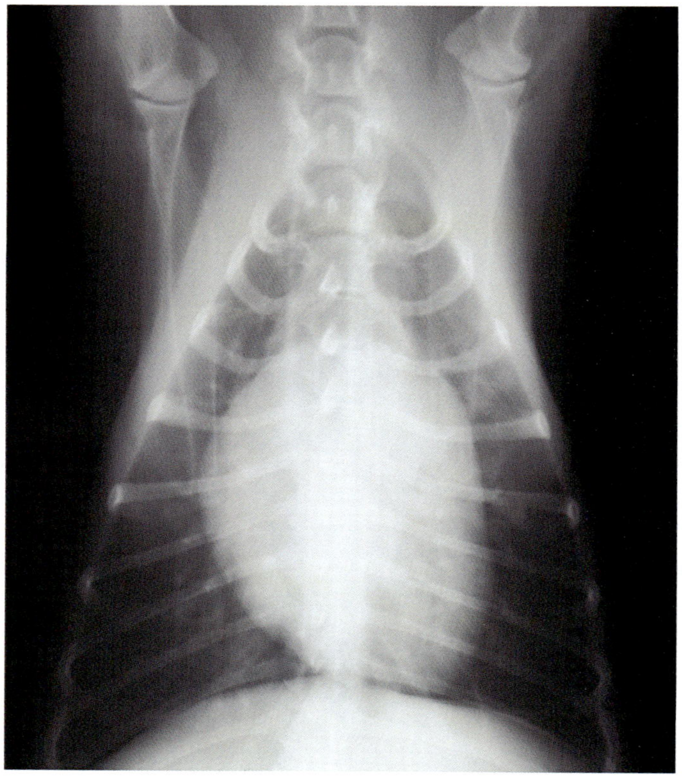

Fig. 22. Ventrodorsal projection of the thorax. The cardiac silhouette is elongated.

To evaluate the conformation of the heart, the side the patient is lying on should be taken into account, because the position of the patient is related to morphological changes in the cardiac silhouette that may lead to diagnostic error. The cardiac silhouette of a patient lying on its right side is egg-shaped, whereas a patient on its left side has a more rounded cardiac silhouette, in which the cardiac apex may appear displaced towards a position slightly dorsal of the sternum. (Figs. 19 and 20).

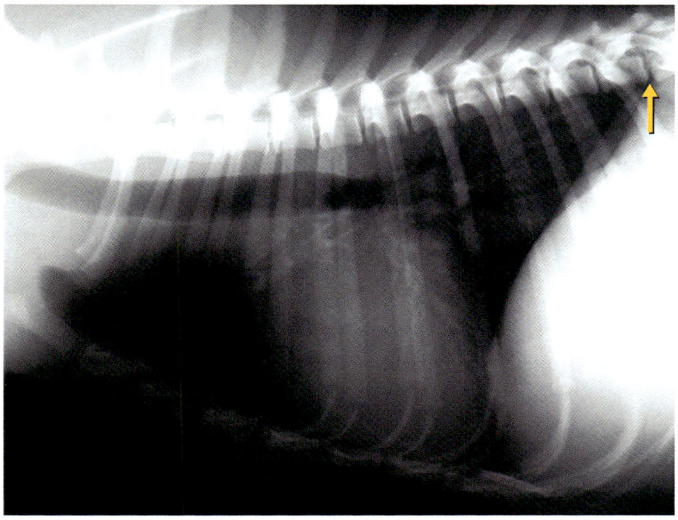

Fig. 23. Radiograph of the thorax during inspiration. The caudodorsal border of the lung (arrow) is situated caudally to the 11th thoracic vertebra T 11.

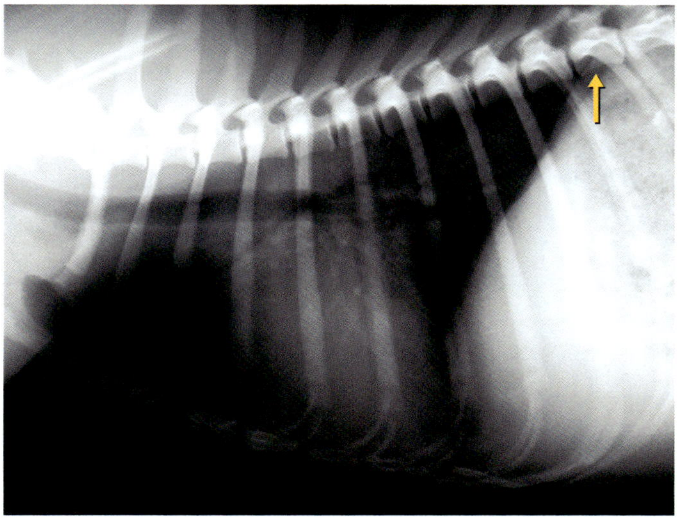

Fig. 24. Radiograph of the lung during exhalation. The caudodorsal border of the lung (arrow) is situated cranially to the 11th thoracic vertebra T 11.

As for the lateral projections, the cardiac silhouette will vary according to whether the **projection is DV or VD**. It appears longer in the ventrodorsal projection, while in dorsoventral projections it has an egg-shape and the cardiac apex is displaced towards the left hemithorax, because the diaphragm has been displaced cranially (Figs. 21 and 22).

The radiograph should be taken **at full inspiration**. On a Lat radiograph at full inspiration, the caudodorsal border of the lung should be caudal to the 11th thoracic vertebra T 11 (Figs. 23 and 24).

In a DV/VD projection, the diaphragmatic dome should be caudal to the centre of T8 and the caudolateral border of the diaphragmatic pulmonary lobes caudal to T 10 (Fig. 25).

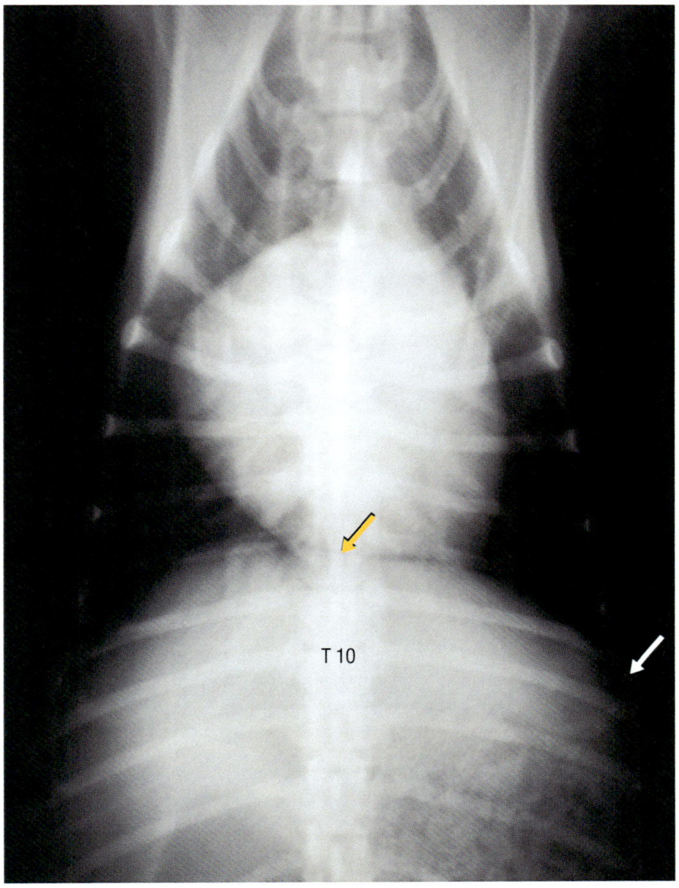

Fig. 25. DV projection of the thorax during inspiration. The diaphragmatic dome appears caudal to the centre of T 8 (yellow arrow) and the caudolateral border of the diaphragmatic lobes appears caudal to T 10 (white arrow).

Lungs

The radiological projections of choice to study the lung parenchyma are the Lat and VD/DV standard projections that have already been described for the thorax.

The following are some comments on the technicalities of pulmonary radiology.

Radiology is an excellent diagnostic tool to evaluate pulmonary abnormalities. This is due to the presence of air (radiolucency) in the lung, which creates a perfect contrast with the soft tissues of the intrathoracic structures and the bony tissues of the extrathoracic structures on the one hand, and with radiopaque lung lesions on the other hand. A fully inflated lung during radiography is crucial for high diagnostic quality of the image.

For a complete radiological evaluation of the lung, three projections should be used: left Lat, right Lat and VD/DV.

Projections in lateral recumbency cause a partial loss of air in the lower lung that is compressed against the table; its radiopacity increases and the contrast with a possible radiopaque lung lesion decreases. For this reason, the uppermost lung provides the best radiographic visualization. When a unilateral lung lesion (for instance, pulmonary metastasis) is suspected, it is therefore advisable to use both right and left lateral projections, as well as the corresponding perpendicular projection.

Visualization of the pulmonary blood vessels

The best visualization of the pulmonary blood vessels is achieved with the patient lying on its left side.

The right cranial lobar blood vessels (artery, vein) and bronchus are in a ventral position in relation to the opacity caused by the craniodorsal mediastinum, while the left side blood vessels are superimposed on the mediastinum. This is why the right cranial lobar artery, bronchus and vein can be used in routine evaluation as a reference for the state of the pulmonary circulation.

Visualization of the right cranial lobar blood vessels is better when the patient is lying on its left, as the right cranial lobe will appear more inflated, which in turn allows a better view of the vessels (Figs. 26 and 27).

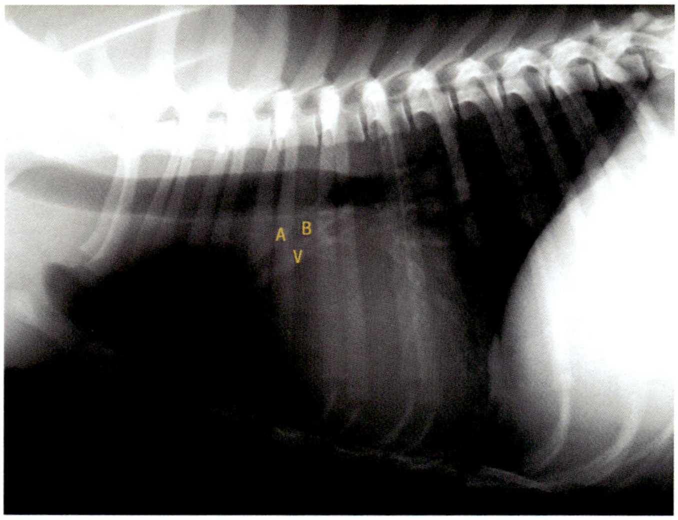

Fig. 26. Left lateral projection of the thorax. There is optimal visualization of the cranial lobar blood vessels of the lung (A: artery, B: bronchus, V: vein).

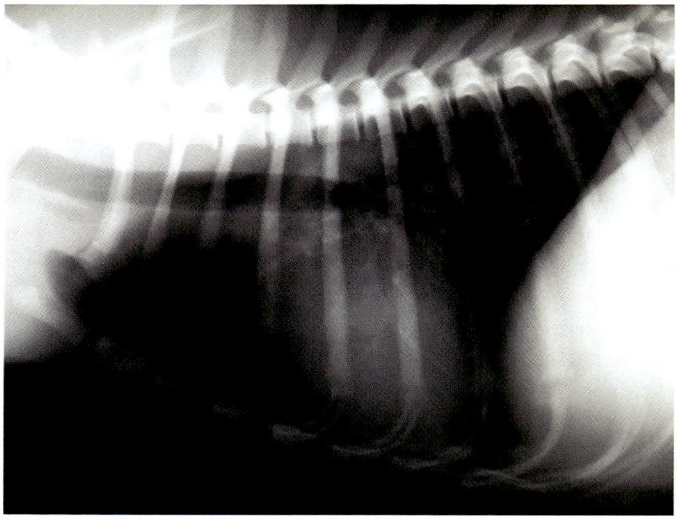

Fig. 27. Right lateral projection of the thorax. Visualization of the cranial lobar blood vessels of the lung is poor.

Visualization of pleural effusion

Small quantities of pleural fluid may go unnoticed on the standard projections Lat and VD/DV if the primary beam does not hit the fluid deposit line tangentially. To ensure a tangential relation between the fluid accumulation and the X-ray beam, a **lateral or ventrodorsal horizontal beam projection of the thorax** can be used. If there is any free pleural fluid, this will gravitate so that the X-ray beam will cross the fluid-gas interface tangentially.

Lateral projection

For lateral horizontal beam projection (Fig. 28):

- Place the patient in sternal or dorsal recumbency.
- Place the cassette as close as possible to the patient, either on the right or the left.
- Pull the forelimbs forward as far as possible.
- Centre the horizontal beam on the thorax.

Ventrodorsal projection

For ventrodorsal horizontal beam projection:

- Place the patient in lateral recumbency, always with the cassette as close as possible to its back.
- Pull the forelimbs forward as far as possible.
- Centre the horizontal beam on the thorax.

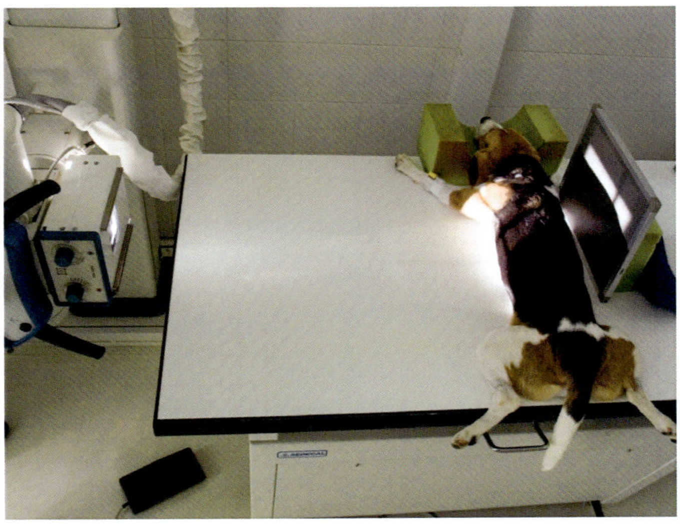

Fig. 28. Lateral projection of the thorax with the patient in sternal recumbency and the primary beam in a horizontal position.

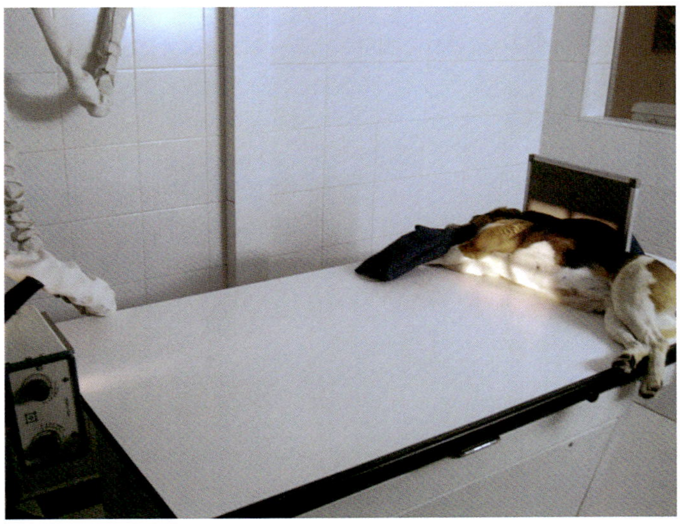

Fig. 29. Ventrodorsal projection of the thorax, with the patient in lateral recumbency and the primary beam in a horizontal position.

Extrathoracic structures

For radiographic examination of the ribs and sternum the standard projections for the thorax are usually satisfactory. However, sometimes it is worthwhile to get additional oblique projections to investigate these structures.

Radiographic examination of the ribs sometimes requires oblique projections.

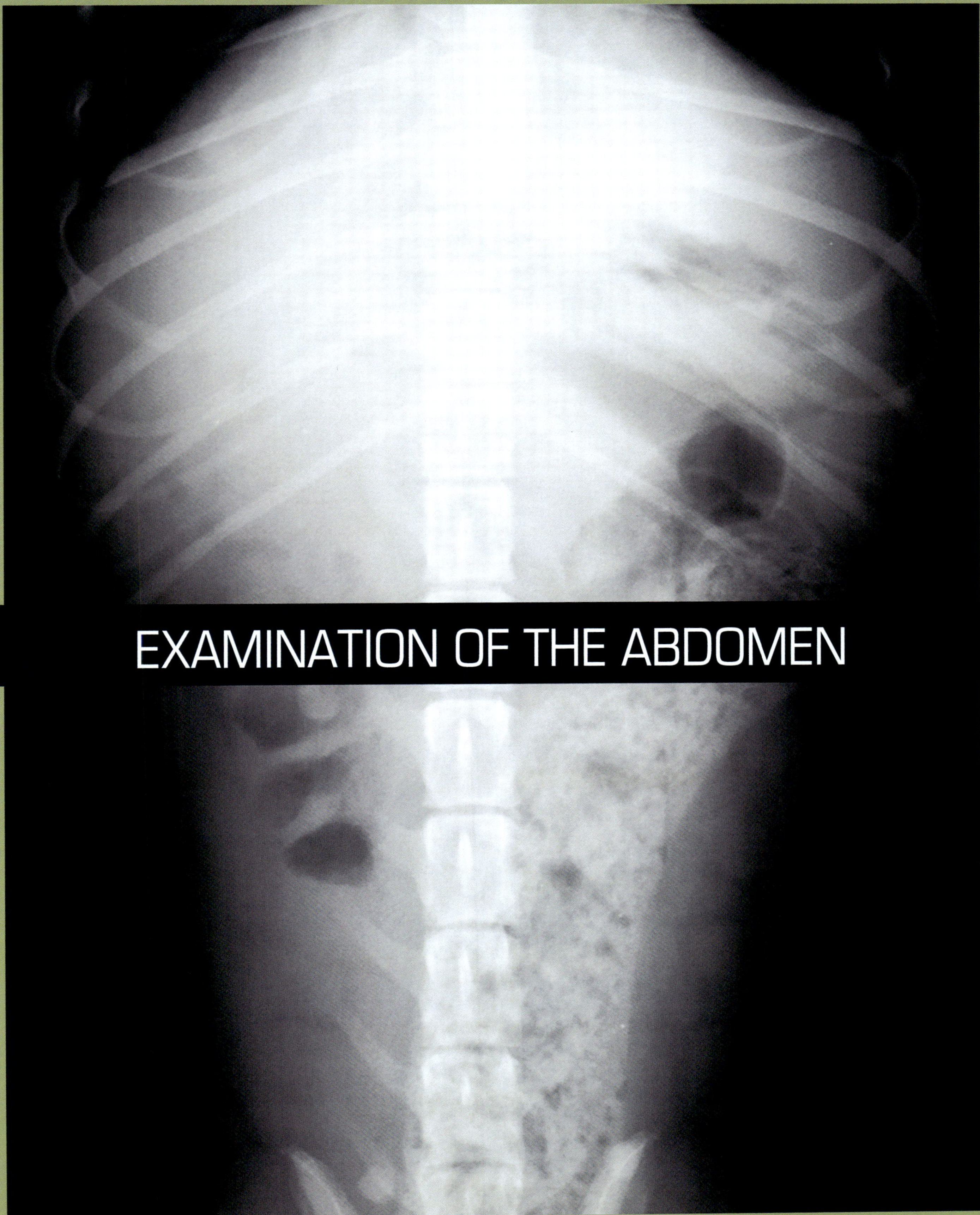

EXAMINATION OF THE ABDOMEN

General considerations

For radiography of the abdomen, it is recommended to use a high milliamperage and a low kilovoltage.

Exposure factors

For routine examination of the abdomen a **high milliamperage-second (mAs)** and a **low kilovoltage (kV)** should be used. The abdomen contains many organs with the same radio-opacity (soft tissue) and the use of a high milliamperage will provide a better definition of these organs.

Positions and projections

Routine radiographic examination of the abdomen requires two perpendicular radiographs. **Preferably, both projections should be performed at expiration** to maximize separation between the different abdominal organs.

One of the projections should be lateral (Lat). It can be carried out with the patient lying either on its left or on its right. When choosing which side, it should be remembered that right lateral recumbency displaces the gas in the stomach and the intestines towards the left side of the animal, i.e. to the gastric fundus and the descending colon, while in left lateral recumbency, the air is displaced towards the right, i.e. to the pylorus and the ascending colon. Hence, the radiological image may differ significantly according to the side that has been chosen, and this should be taken into account during radiological interpretation.

Right lateral recumbency causes displacement of digestive gas towards the gastric fundus and the descending colon, whereas in left lateral recumbency, it is displaced towards the pylorus and the ascending colon.

For the **lateral (Lat) projection** of the abdomen (Figs. 1 and 2):

- Place the patient in lateral recumbency on the side of choice and ensure that the spinal column is parallel to the tabletop, as an oblique positioning of the patient may lead to an incorrect radiological diagnosis.
- Keep the head in slight extension.
- Pull the forelimbs forward and the hind limbs backward.
- Centre the X-ray beam on the last rib for examination of the cranial abdomen and on the middle of the abdomen to examine the caudal part.

In the selection of exposure factors, it should be remembered that the cranial abdomen is thicker than the caudal part, so that, in general, the kilovoltage should be set 4 kV higher for examination of the organs in the cranial abdomen.

- The complete abdomen should be included.
- Wait for full expiration to take the radiograph.

Examination of the cranial abdomen requires an increase of 4 kV as compared to the caudal part.

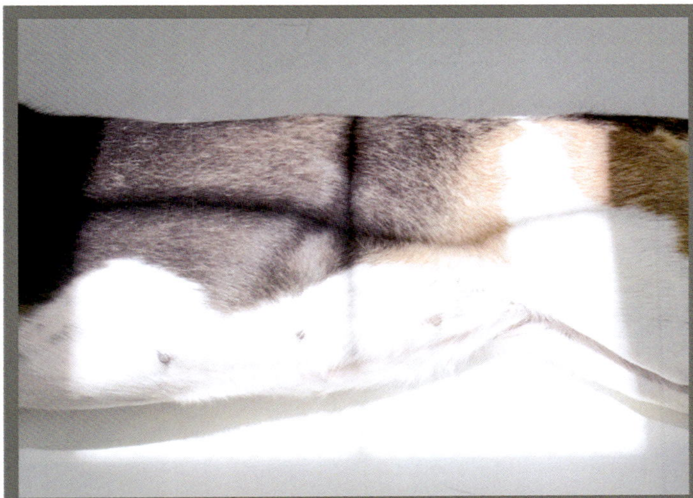

Fig. 1. Patient in lateral recumbency for lateral projection of the abdomen.

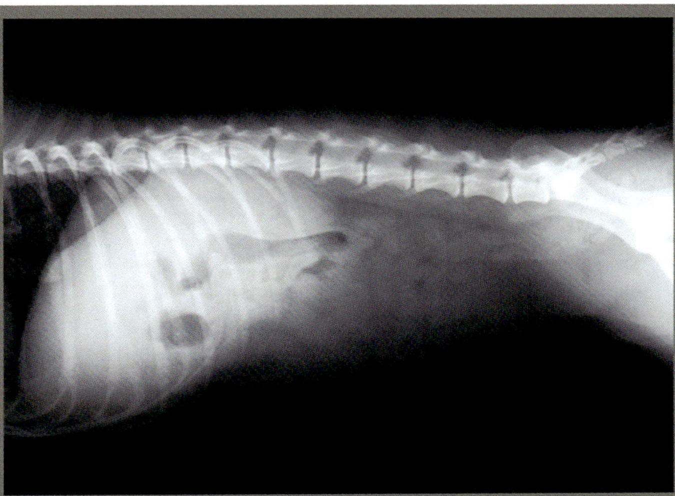

Fig. 2. Lat projection of the abdomen.

After the lateral projection, a perpendicular image should be obtained: either the dorsoventral (DV) or the ventrodorsal (VD) projection. The dorsoventral projection allows a more natural distribution of the abdominal viscera, but some animals resist this position, in which case the ventrodorsal position can be used. As in the Lat projection, the distribution of gas in the digestive tract will vary according to the position of the patient; sternal recumbency (DV projection) favours air movement towards the gastric fundus and the transverse colon, while in dorsal recumbency (VD projection) air moves towards the pylorus and descending colon.

In the DV projection, digestive gas is displaced towards the gastric fundus and the transverse colon, while in the VD projection it moves towards the pylorus and the descending colon.

For the **dorsoventral projection (DV)** (Figs. 3 and 4):

- Place the patient in sternal recumbency. To avoid rotation of the body, foam wedges can be placed on both sides of the abdomen.
- Keep the head on the table in a natural position.
- Pull the forelimbs forward and the hind limbs backward.
- Centre the X-ray beam at the level of the last rib.
- The complete abdomen should be included.
- Wait for full expiration to take the radiograph.

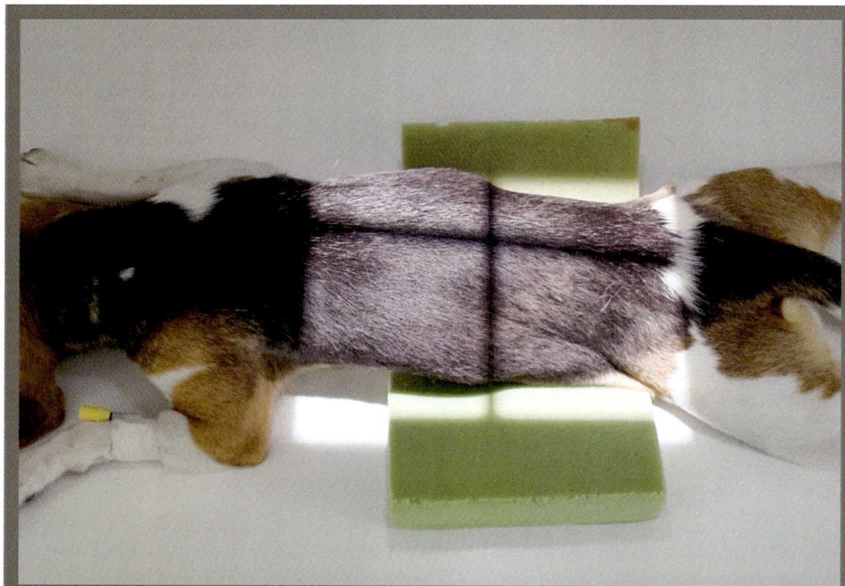

Fig. 3. Animal in sternal recumbency for the dorsoventral projection.

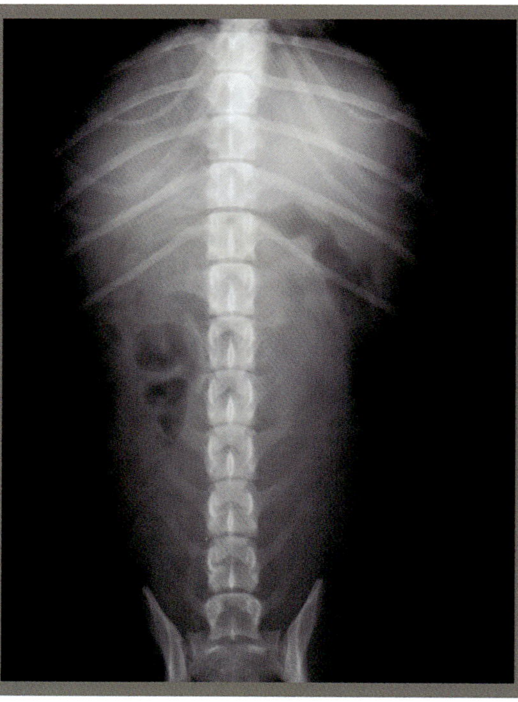

Fig. 4. DV projection of the abdomen. ▶

For the **ventrodorsal projection (VD)** (Figs. 5 and 6):

- Place the patient in dorsal recumbency.
- Keep the head in a neutral position.
- Pull the forelimbs forward and the hind limbs backward.
- Centre the X-ray beam at the level of the last rib.
- The complete abdomen should be included.
- Wait for full expiration to take the radiograph.
- In the VD projection the kilovoltage should be reduced by about 10% compared to the DV projection.

The VD projection requires a 10% reduction in kilovoltage compared to the DV projection.

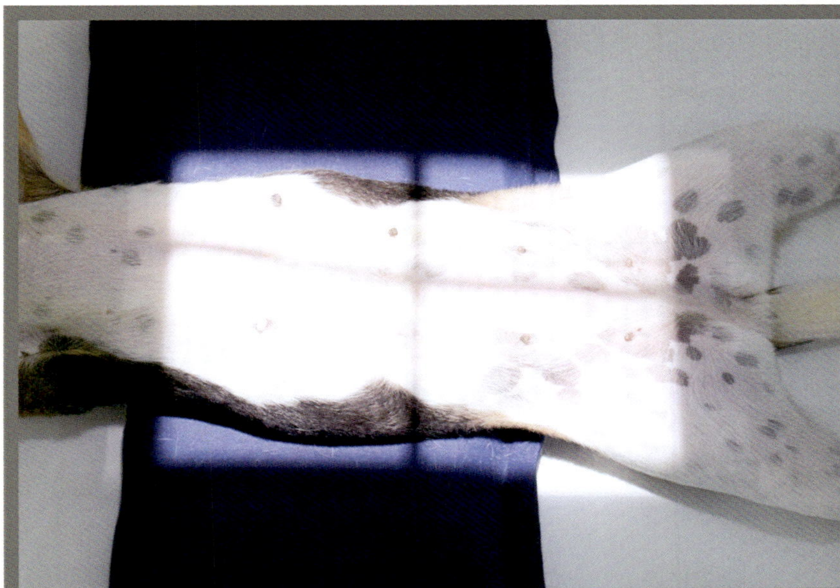

Fig. 5. Animal in dorsal recumbency for the ventrodorsal projection.

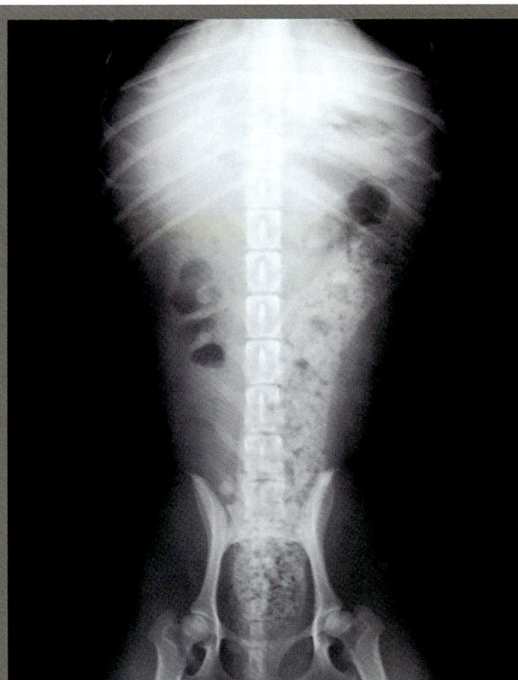

Fig. 6. VD projection of the abdomen. ▶

Liver and spleen

Routine radiological examination of the liver and spleen requires the use of the standard projections Lat and VD/DV already described. These projections provide information on the position, size, shape, outline and radiopacity of these two organs. However, it should be kept in mind that radiology does not provide information on focal or diffuse alterations of the parenchyma, so that it is often necessary to complement the radiological examination with an ultrasound scan.

Kidneys and ureters

The standard abdominal Lat and VD/DV projections that have been described provide information on the size, shape, position and radiopacity of the kidneys. However, to examine the parenchyma and functionality, an ultrasound scan and/or a radiological contrast technique are required (excretion urography).

Normal ureters cannot be visualized with plain radiography; excretion urography is the best technique to examine them.

Excretion urography

Excretion urography is useful to investigate the structure and functionality of the kidneys and ureters. This technique consists of administering a positive contrast medium by intravenous injection, which will cause sequential opacification of the kidneys, ureters and urinary bladder, according to the kidneys' capacity to concentrate and excrete the medium.

Excretion urography requires the use of an iodinated contrast medium.

The positive contrast medium used for urography has to be iodinated. Usually, the use of a ionic iodinated agent is satisfactory (e.g. sodium amidotrizoate) except in high-risk patients, when it is recommended that a non-ionic iodinated contrast medium is used (iohexol or iopamidol).

The recommended dose for the contrast medium is 450-880 mg of the iodinated complex/kg bodyweight.

Recommendations for excretion urography:

- **Preparation of the patient**: to obtain the best possible radiographic visualization of the kidneys and ureters, it is essential that the digestive tract is empty. Food should be withheld for 24 hours and it is also advisable to administer rectal enemas 12 and 3 hours before the examination.
- **Catheterisation of the cephalic or jugular vein**. If necessary the animal should be tranquillised or anaesthetised.

- **Plain abdominal radiographs in standard projections Lat and VD**. It should be emphasised that the right lateral projection is more suitable than the left, because it allows better longitudinal separation between the right and the left kidney, which may facilitate radiological interpretation.
- **Bolus injection of the contrast medium** of choice through the catheter.
- **Sequential radiographic projections** at approximately the following intervals:

The right lateral projection is more suitable than the left for excretion urography, as it allows better longitudinal separation between the right and the left kidney.

- Straight after injection of the contrast medium (VD projection).
- 15 seconds after injection (VD projection).
- 5 minutes after injection (VD, Lat and oblique projections).
- 15 minutes after injection (VD and Lat projections).
- 30 minutes after injection (VD and Lat projections).

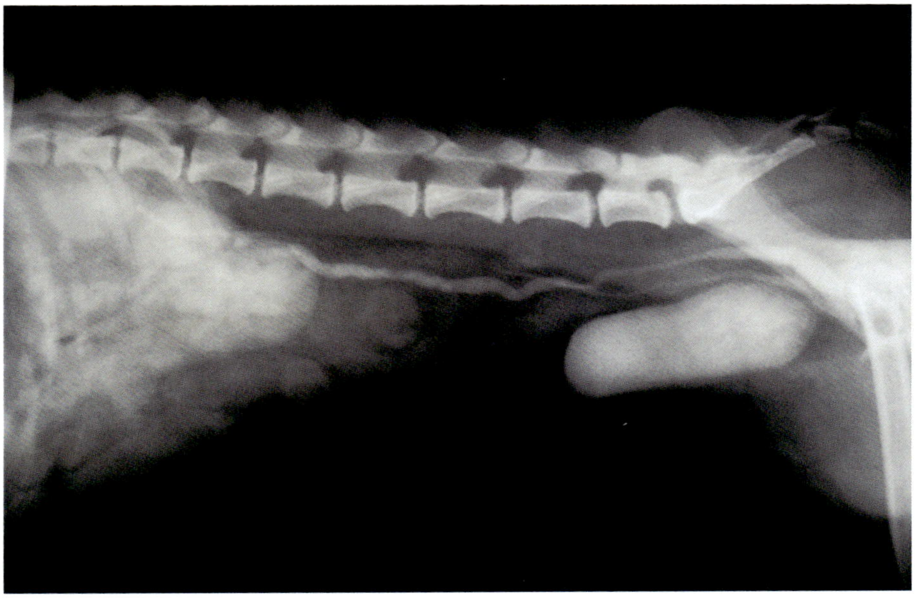

Fig. 7. Excretion urography. Lat projection 5 minutes after injection of the contrast medium. Ectopic ureters can be observed.

If the patient suffers from renal insufficiency, it may be necessary to increase the dose of the contrast medium.

It should be remembered that visualization of renal opacification after injection of the contrast medium depends on renal function: the poorer the functionality, the less opacification will occur. For this reason, both the dose of contrast medium and the exposure intervals should be adapted to each particular case (Fig. 7).

Urinary bladder

The lateral and ventrodorsal projections of the caudal abdomen may provide information on the position, shape, size and radiopacity of the bladder. However, if plain radiography suggests bladder disease and a more exhaustive study is required, a radiographic contrast study may be called for (contrast cystography).

Retrograde contrast cystography

This is a radiological contrast technique in which a positive contrast medium (positive cystography), a negative contrast medium (pneumocystography) or a combination of the two (double contrast cystography) are injected into the urinary bladder via a urethral catheter.

Positive cystography is the radiological technique of choice to locate the position of the urinary bladder. The positive contrast medium should be iodinated, but an ionic complex may be used (e.g. meglumine or sodium amidotrizoate), at a dose of 10 ml per kilogram bodyweight.

Pneumocystography is the technique of choice when trying to optimise visualization of radiopaque uroliths. In this case, the most commonly used contrast medium is 10 to 100 ml of air, according to the size of the patient; it is advisable to palpate the bladder through the abdominal wall during injection to prevent over distension.

Double contrast cystography is the technique of choice to demonstrate alterations in the vesical mucous membranes.

While injecting the contrast medium for a cystography, it is advisable to palpate the bladder through the abdominal wall to prevent over distension.

Recommendations for retrograde contrast cystography:

- **Preparation of the patient**: to obtain the best possible radiographic visualization of the bladder, it is essential that the digestive tract is empty of faecal contents. Food should be withheld for 24 hours and it is also advisable to administer a rectal enema before the examination.
- **Urethral catheter**. If necessary tranquillise or anaesthetise the patient.
- **Emptying the urinary bladder**.
- **Positive cystography**: with a syringe, inject the positive contrast medium (iodinated) through the urethral catheter, while palpating the bladder continuously through the abdominal wall. If the bladder is felt to be sufficiently distended or return pressure is felt on the plunger of the syringe before the full estimated dose of the contrast medium has been injected, the injection should be stopped.

  Once the medium has been injected, the bladder is massaged carefully to aid in its distribution.

If possible, three different radiological projections of the caudal abdomen should be obtained: lateral (Fig. 8), ventrodorsal and oblique ventrodorsal. The latter avoids superimposition of the bladder on the vertebral column, making visualization easier.

- **Double contrast cystography**: Once the radiographic images of the positive contrast cystography have been obtained, as much urine as possible is removed from the bladder, and the negative contrast (air) is injected, remembering to palpate the bladder through the abdominal wall to prevent over distension. If possible, three different radiological projections of the caudal abdomen should be obtained: lateral (Fig. 9), ventrodorsal and oblique ventrodorsal.

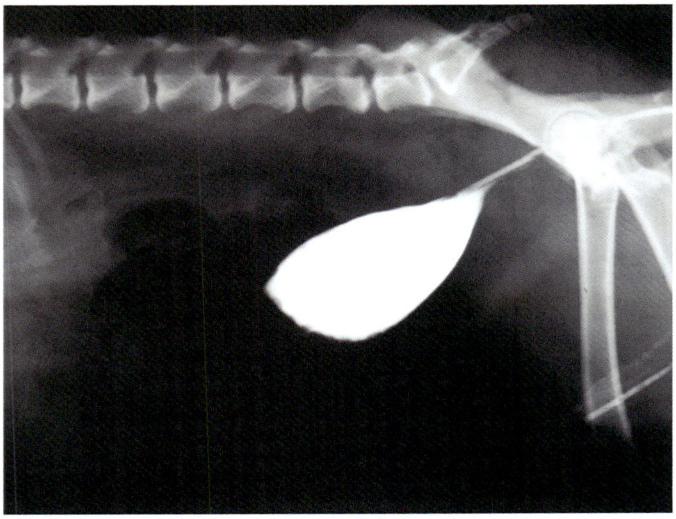

Fig. 8. Positive contrast cystography. Lat projection.

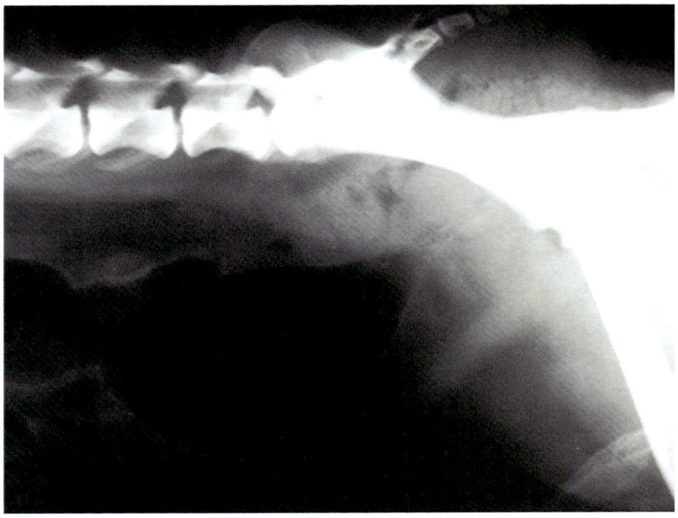

Fig. 9. Double contrast cystography. Lat projection.

Even though the contrast techniques for examination of the bladder are not very complicated, some common mistakes may lead to radiological artefacts that make interpretation difficult.

The **most common artefacts** are seen during positive contrast cystography and are caused by air bubbles in the bladder and/or false filling defects. Air bubbles give rise to intra-luminal filling defects of the bladder, which may simulate a thickening of the vesical wall or the presence of radiolucent uroliths. To avoid air bubbles, no air should be allowed into the urethral catheter at any time; a three way tap connected to the catheter may be of help, as it permits the injection of the positive contrast medium immediately after having emptied the bladder.

It is also possible to mistakenly diagnose filling defects of the bladder (and even mistake them for neoplasia), which is why it is essential to achieve adequate distension of the bladder with the positive contrast medium.

To avoid air bubbles during positive cystography, a three-way tap connected to the urethral catheter can be of help.

Urethra

Examination of the urethra is very common in male animals, while it is almost never required in females.

Sometimes the presence of radiopaque uroliths shows up during plain radiography. However, if urethral abnormalities are suspected, it is advisable to add a positive contrast study (contrast urethrography).

For plain radiological examination of the urethra (Figs. 10 and 11):

- Place the patient in lateral recumbency, with the forelimbs pulled cranially and the hind limbs pulled cranially too, to avoid superimposition of the femurs on the urethra.
- Remove the tail from the X-ray field.
- Centre the X-ray beam at the level of the ischium and collimate, including the penile bone.

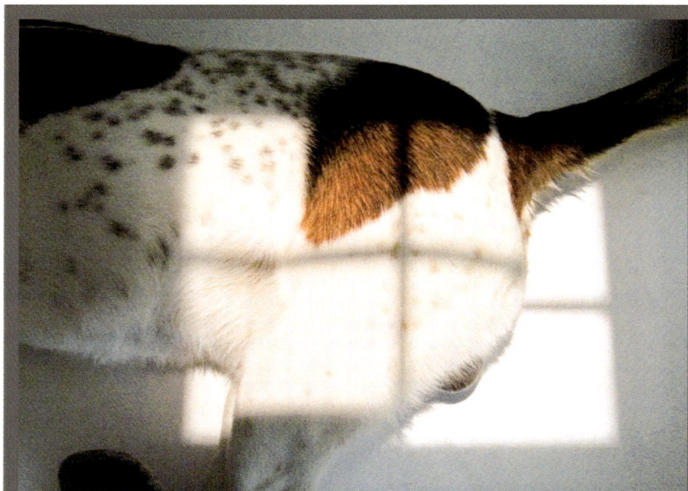

Fig. 10. Positioning of the animal to examine the urethra.

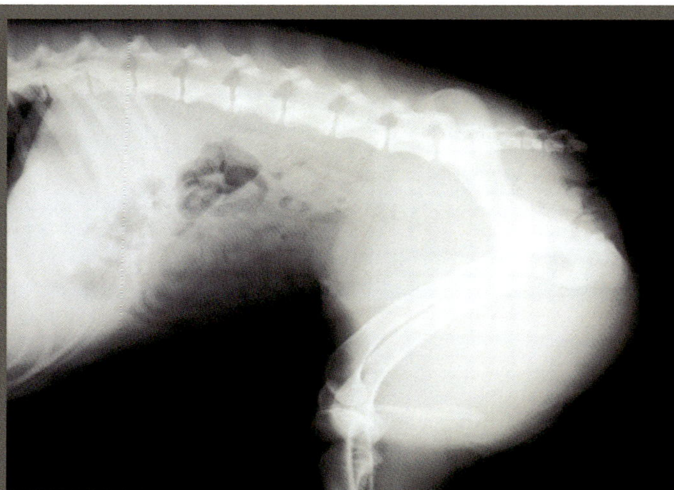

Fig. 11. The position allows radiographic examination of the complete course of the urethra.

Contrast urethrography

This is a radiological technique where positive contrast medium is introduced into the urethra. It should be an iodinated medium, although there is no need for it to be non-ionic. The recommended dose in dogs varies between 10 and 15 ml.

For this technique, a urethral catheter should be introduced approximately 10 cm into the urethra. With the animal in lateral recumbency and the hind limbs pulled cranially, the contrast medium is injected into the catheter until there is 1-2 ml of the estimated volume left; this is the moment the radiograph should be taken (Fig. 12). To avoid air bubbles, which may cause unwelcome artefacts, it is recommended to fill the catheter with sterile saline solution before injecting the column of contrast medium.

To avoid air bubbles in a contrast urethrography, it is recommended to fill the catheter with sterile saline solution before injecting the positive contrast medium.

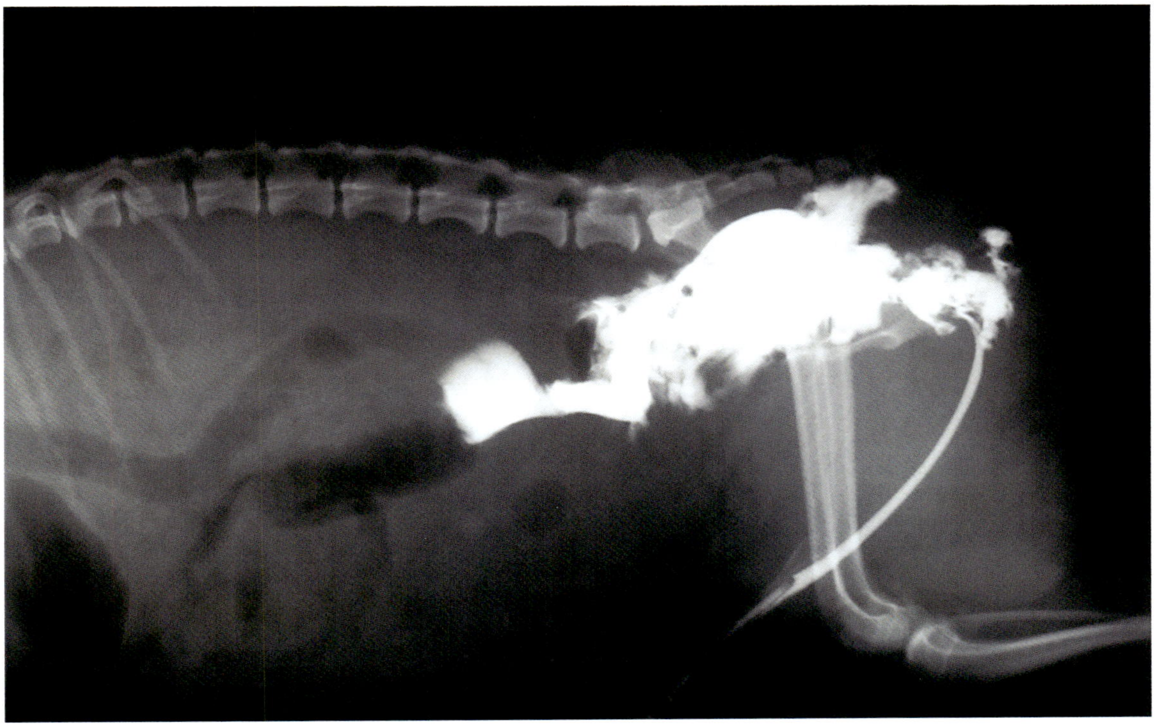

Fig. 12. Positive urethrography. The technique demonstrates rupture of the urethra.

Stomach and small intestine

Routine examination of the stomach and small intestine requires the use of the lateral and dorsoventral/ventrodorsal abdominal projections described at the start of this chapter.

Stomach

A complete radiological examination of the stomach requires four projections: right lateral, left lateral, dorsoventral and ventrodorsal. As described in the general considerations in this chapter, it is important to remember that the position of the patient during radiography will determine the position of the stomach and thus the internal distribution of its contents (gas-liquid). This should be kept in mind for a correct interpretation of the radiographs.

On many occasions, plain radiography of the stomach is not sufficient to reach a diagnosis and a radiographic contrast study or gastrography is called for (see the section on digestive contrast study on this page). However, the benefits of a gastrography often do not offset the cost to the clinician, which is why, when a "pure" gastric abnormality is suspected, it is recommended to perform an ultrasound scan and /or endoscopy of the stomach.

Small intestine

Plain radiography of the small intestine (lateral and ventrodorsal standard projections) may provide valuable diagnostic information on its shape, size, outline, position and radiopacity. However, assessment of mucosal alterations, peristalsis and intestinal transit time require the use of radiclogical contrast techniques and/or ultrasound/endoscopy.

Contrast study of the upper digestive tract

This radiographic technique consists of the oral administration of a positive contrast medium to examine the upper digestive tract by radiological opacification.

Recommendations for a contrast study of the upper digestive tract:

- **Preparation of the patient**: whenever possible, the patient should be prepared by withholding the food for 24 hours and an enema should be given 4 hours before radiographic examination. However, the majority of disorders that require a contrast study are acute cases and proper preparation of the patient is therefore impossible.

- **Contrast medium**. The contrast medium used in this type of radiographic examination should be positive. The most commonly used medium is barium sulphate suspension. Its main advantages are its low cost and high radiopacity, which provides good definition of the intestinal mucosa. However, its use is completely contraindicated when gastrointestinal perforation is suspected, because it is extremely irritant to the tissues of the peritoneal cavity. Hence an iodinated contrast medium, which is not irritant to the peritoneal cavity, should be used when perforation is suspected.

When intestinal perforation is suspected, an iodinated contrast medium should be used instead of barium.

However, iodinated agents have several disadvantages. For one, they are less radiopaque than barium sulphate, so they provide less diagnostic information. Also, affordable iodinated agents in veterinary medicine are ionic (sodium and meglumine amidotrizoate) and these agents are hypertonic. Their hypertonicity causes liquid to flow into the intestinal tract, and this should be remembered in hypovolemic patients, whose state of dehydration may worsen.

Non-ionic iodinated agents do not have this disadvantage, but are very expensive.

Another positive contrast medium used for radiographic studies of the digestive tract are barium-impregnated polyethylene spheres (BIPS). These spheres are useful for assessment of digestive transit time (in particular to detect obstructions); however, they do not provide information on the mucous membranes of the tract.

When carrying out a gastrointestinal contrast study, it should also be remembered that there is a **direct relation between the type and amount of contrast medium used and the digestive transit time**. The iodinated contrast media pass much more quickly through the digestive tract than barium sulphate.

The use of ionic iodinated agents in dehydrated animals should be avoided.

The amount of contrast medium will also affect digestive transit time and it is likely that an incorrect dose is the most important cause of diagnostic errors when using this technique. The recommended doses for the different contrast media are shown in table I.

The use of an inadequate dose of contrast medium leads to many diagnostic errors.

Table I. Dose for contrast media used for examination of the gastrointestinal tract.

	Barium sulphate suspension	Ionic iodinated agents
Dog	6-10 ml/kg	2-3 ml/kg

- **Administration of the contrast medium**. The contrast medium for examination of the digestive tract is administered orally. The medium of choice can be administered with a syringe, an orogastric tube or it can be mixed with food.
  In docile patients, the barium sulphate may be administered with a small syringe. Do not forget to cover the animal's coat with a protective bib to avoid positive contrast agent staining, which will show up in the radiograph as an artefact (Fig. 13).

Care should be taken to avoid accidental aspiration during oral administration of barium contrast medium with a syringe.

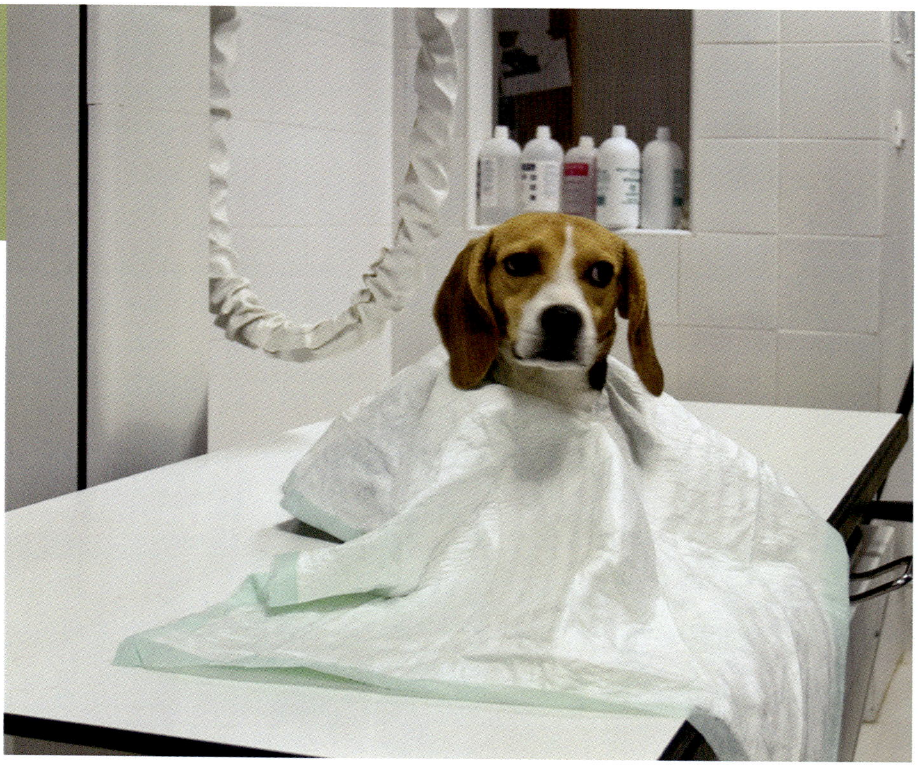

Fig. 13. Before administering the positive contrast medium, the animal should be covered with a bib.

Care should be taken when administering the barium agent, as it may be accidentally inhaled into the respiratory tract, where it cannot be reabsorbed.

In patients that are difficult to handle, where there is greater risk of inhalation, it is preferable to use an iodinated agent, as this will be reabsorbed easily. If the sedation of these patients is required, it should be remembered that many drugs have an effect on gastrointestinal motility.

Contrast media can also be mixed with food, although in this case it should be remembered that the amount and type of gastric contents will also have an influence on digestive transit time.

- **Sequential radiological standard projections** (lateral and ventrodorsal) (Fig. 14), taking into account that the different parts of the digestive tract will become radiopaque at different times, according to the contrast agent used, as shown in table II.

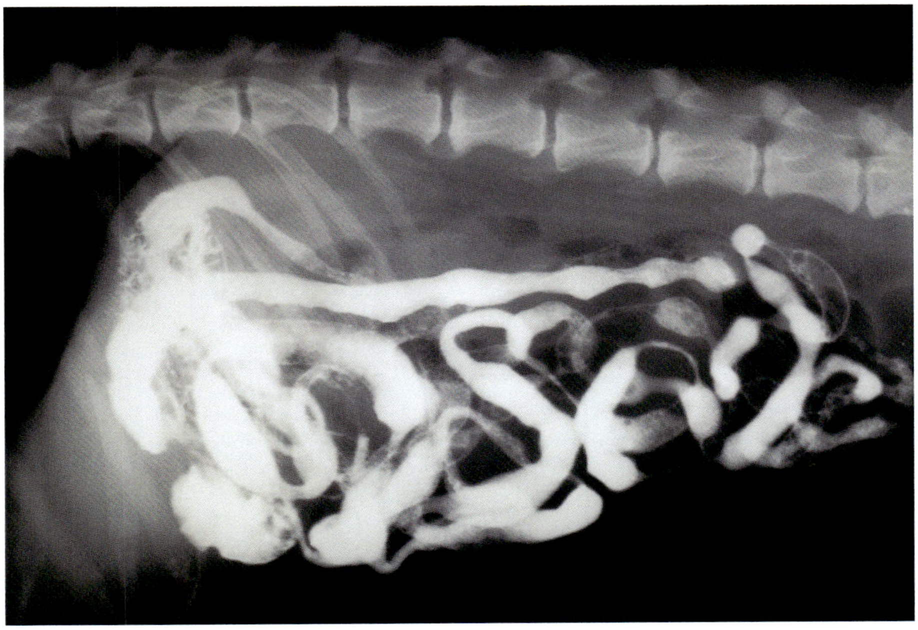
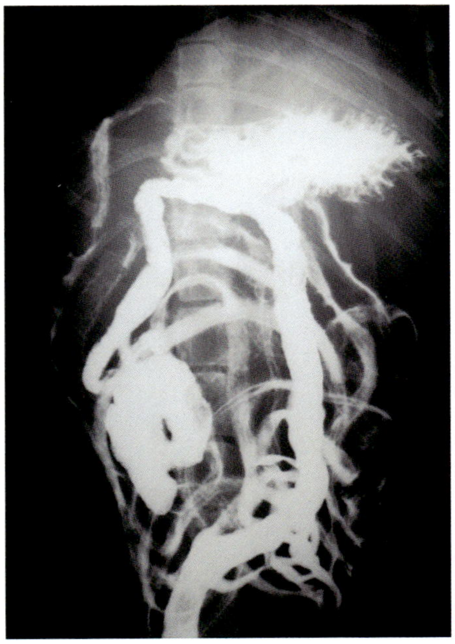

Fig. 14. Digestive transit. Lat and VD projection.

Table II: Interval until opacification of the digestive tract in the dog.

	Stomach	Duodenum	Jejunum	Entire small intestine	Colon
Barium	Zero time	15 minutes	1 hour	2 hours	4 hours
Iodine	Zero time	——	15 minutes	30 minutes	1 hour

Large intestine

Basic radiographic examination of the large intestine requires the standard projections Lat and VD for the complete abdomen as described at the start of this chapter. However, on many occasions, plain radiography does not provide sufficient diagnostic information and a contrast study with a positive agent (barium enema), air (pneumocolonography) or a combination of both (double contrast study) is called for. Nowadays, contrast techniques have been superseded by more sensitive diagnostic techniques such as ultrasonography or endoscopy.

Colonography

This is the contrast technique for examination of the large intestine.

Recommendations for colonography:

- **Preparation of the patient**. To ensure that the large intestine does not contain faecal matter, food should be withheld for 24 hours before the study. Also, oral laxatives should be given and a rectal enema should be administered before radiographic examination.
- **Anaesthesia of the patient**.
- **Administration of the contrast medium (barium enema)**. The most commonly used agent for examination of the large intestine is a barium sulphate suspension which is administered through a tube (equipped with an inflatable cuff to avoid reflux) that has been inserted in the distal part of the rectum. The dose of barium varies from 7 to 15 ml/kg bodyweight, although it is advisable to monitor administration radiographically until the desired effect is achieved. It should be remembered that the use of barium should be avoided when intestinal perforation is suspected (irritant to the peritoneal cavity); it should be substituted for an iodinated agent.
- **Radiographic exposure** (Fig. 15). Once there is adequate distension of the colon, left lateral, ventrodorsal and oblique (right ventral - left dorsal and left ventral - right dorsal) projections should be obtained.
- **Double contrast**. If a double contrast study is required, as much of the barium as possible should be removed, air introduced and the same radiographic projections repeated.

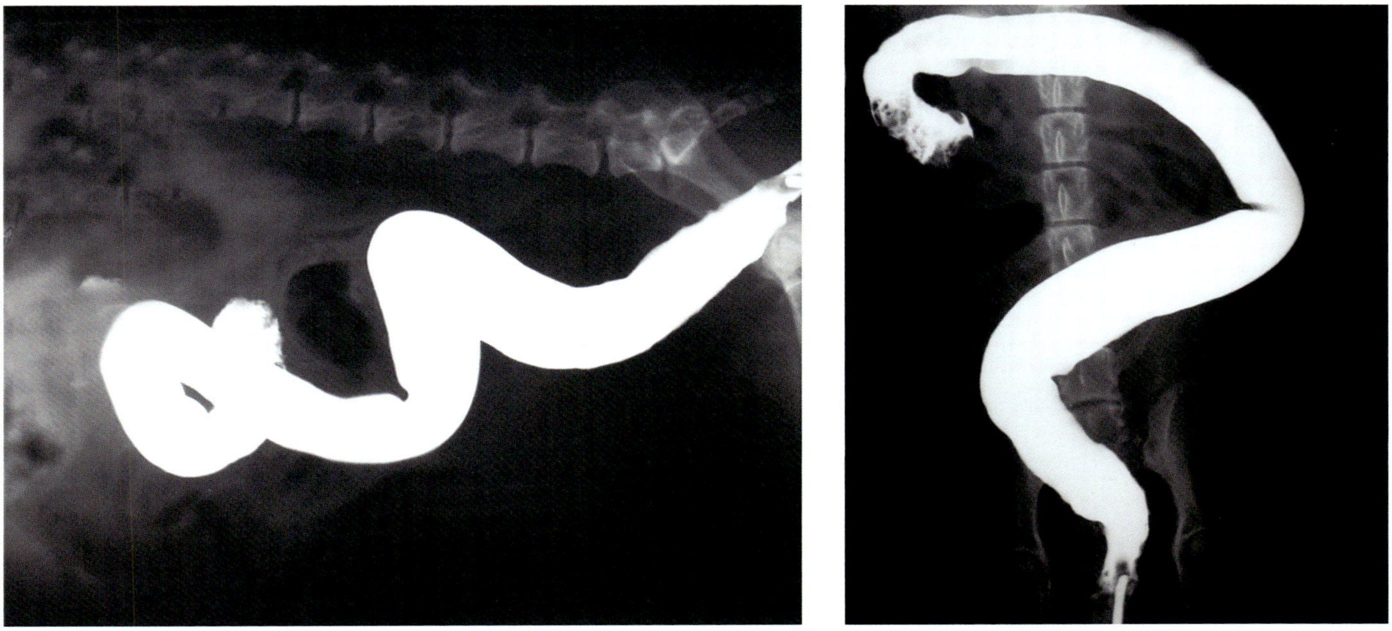

Fig. 15. Barium enema, lateral and VD projections.

Diaphragm

Examination of the diaphragm requires the standard projections Lat and VD/DV described in the general considerations. However, on many occasions, the radiographic images obtained with these projections are not sufficient to reach a diagnostic verdict on the most common diaphragmatic disorder in dogs: diaphragmatic hernia.

In that case a radiographic contrast technique, positive peritoneography, is called for.

A positive peritoneography may be decisive for a radiological diagnosis of diaphragmatic hernia.

Positive peritoneography or celiography

This is a simple radiographic technique that consists of the introduction of positive contrast medium in the peritoneal cavity. Recommendations:

- **Preparation of the patient**: it is advisable to withhold the food for 24 hours to ensure that the gastrointestinal tract is empty, although this is not essential.
- **Anaesthesia of the patient** is advisable.
- **Cleaning and disinfection of the puncture site**: the midpoint between the umbilical area and the pubis.

- **Insert the catheter** through the abdominal wall into the peritoneal cavity and aspirate with a syringe to ensure that no organ or abdominal vessel has been punctured.
- **Inject a small amount of iodinated positive contrast medium** and take a radiograph in lateral projection during injection to ensure that the catheter is in the correct place.
- **Inject** 20-30 ml of the contrast medium. Even though it is more expensive, it is recommended to use a non-ionic agent.
- **Roll** the animal over to ensure the even distribution of the medium through the whole peritoneal cavity.
- **Radiographic exposures**. The radiographic projection should be chosen according to the suspected problem. In general, the right and left Lat and VD/DV abdominal standard projections described previously should be used.

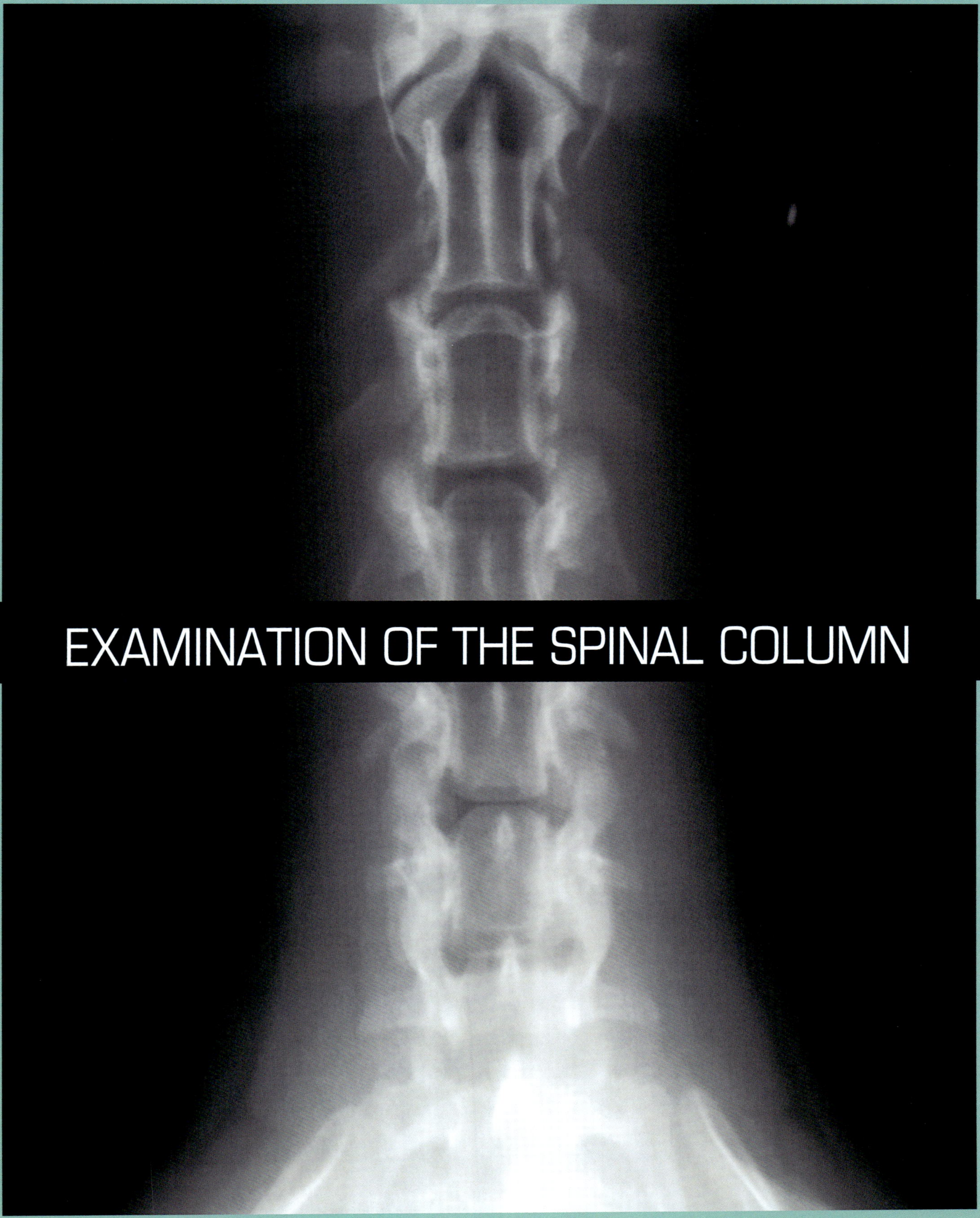

EXAMINATION OF THE SPINAL COLUMN

General considerations

For correct positioning and a good examination of the spinal column, it is necessary to, at least, **sedate** the patient, and sometimes use **general anaesthesia**; especially if myelography or spinal surgery are to take place. The reason is that most radiological examinations of the spine are very painful and provoke involuntary muscular contraction, which leads to incorrect positioning of the patient.

A correct position is always essential to establish a correct radiological diagnosis, and in the case of the spinal column, an incorrect position makes it very difficult to assess: whether the intervertebral spaces and foramina are similar in shape and size (when looking for herniation of a disk), the adjacent vertebrae have normal size and shape (vertebral malformations) or if the vertebrae have the expected radiological density (vertebral neoplasia or systemic disease).

It is advisable to have foam wedges of different shapes and sizes to hand, which can be used to avoid positioning defects in the different sections of the spinal column.

Utmost care should be taken during positioning when a spinal fracture or instability is suspected, as the lesion may get worse or even become irreversible when forced positions, i.e. forced flexion or extension, are used.

> Forced positions of the spine should be handled gently, otherwise lesions may become irreversible.

Exposure factors

Radiological examination of the spinal column requires the use of a **low kilovoltage (kV) and a high milliamperage-second (mAs)**. This will result in a very short grey scale, which provides adequate contrast between the bone and the soft tissue.

It is advisable to use rare-earth screens, and, except for cats and very small dogs, an anti-scatter grid should be used to reduce scattered radiation.

Positions and projections

Radiographic investigation of the spinal column requires two perpendicular radiographs: lateral (Lat) and ventrodorsal (VD) (or on occasion DV).

For the lateral projection, it makes no difference whether the patient is on its right or left side, as the radiographic anatomy is the same. The authors prefer to standardize their method and use, whenever possible, **right lateral recumbency**.

In VD projection, the distance between the object and the film is reduced, which improves definition. In cases of herniation of the disk and myelography, it is also very useful to make a decision on the surgical approach to the lesion. For the cervical column an additional special position is discussed.

The spinal column should always be perfectly parallel to the X-ray table, as any positioning defect will make it very difficult to establish a good radiological diagnosis. Aids for perfect positioning include radiolucent foam pieces of different shapes mentioned previously, which do not interfere with interpretation, and sandbags that help to attain a perfect right angle between X-ray beam and patient, especially in radiographs in VD projection.

Cervical column

Radiological examination of the cervical column presents certain difficulties, because this is the most mobile and flexible area of the whole column. Furthermore, it is bordered by two structures that are relatively voluminous when the patient is lying on the X-ray table: the head and the thoracic inlet.

Recommendations for the **lateral (Lat) projection**:

- Place the patient in lateral recumbency, generally on its right side, with the vertebral column parallel to the tabletop.
- To maintain this position, a foam wedge should be placed between the table and the animal's neck, at approximately C3-C4.
- Depending on the breed and the size of the head, it is often necessary to place a foam aid under the muzzle too, to avoid rotation due to the smaller volume of this area.
- It is advisable to place a rectangular foam piece between the forelegs to keep them in a parallel position and avoid axial rotation.
- The forelegs should be pulled **caudally**, especially when investigating the caudal cervical column, to avoid the soft tissues of the legs and shoulders overlying the area under study. **Cranial** traction with a bandage or a string should be exerted on the mandible and maxilla, so that the true size of the intervertebral disk spaces can be visualized.
- For a complete investigation of the cervical column it is best to take two radiographs, centred on C2-C3 and C5-C6.

- If **vertebral instability** is suspected, for instance in cases of atlanto-axial subluxation or vertebral fracture or dislocation, it may be necessary to use stress or forced positions, with the column in flexion or extension; however, the column should never be forced excessively, as the clinical signs of cord compression may be exacerbated by this manoeuvre.

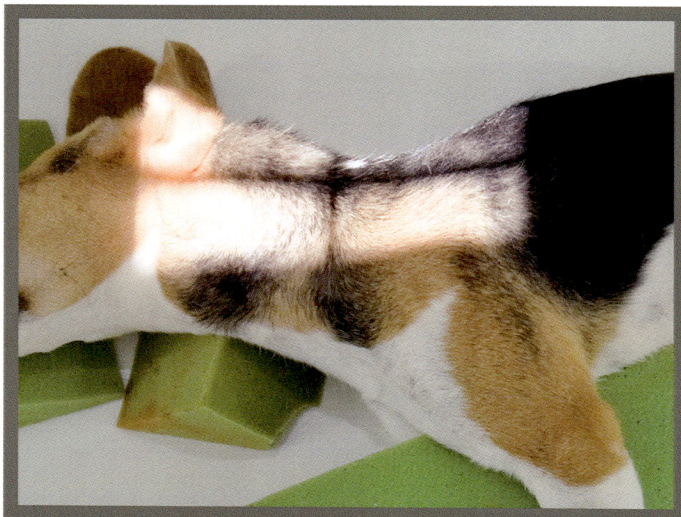

Fig. 1. Patient in the correct position for lateral projection of the cervical column.

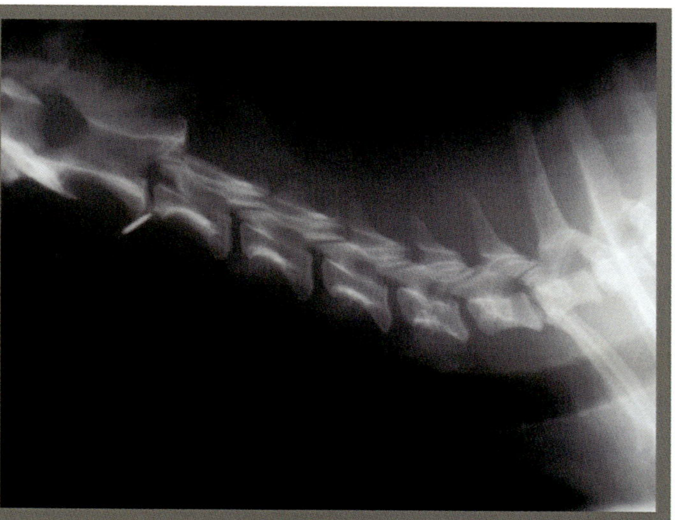

Fig. 2. Radiograph of a well-positioned cervical column in figure 1.

If all these points are taken into account, an image like the one in figure 2 will be obtained. It is very different from figure 3, in which it is impossible to assess alterations in the area, because neither traction nor foam wedges have been used.

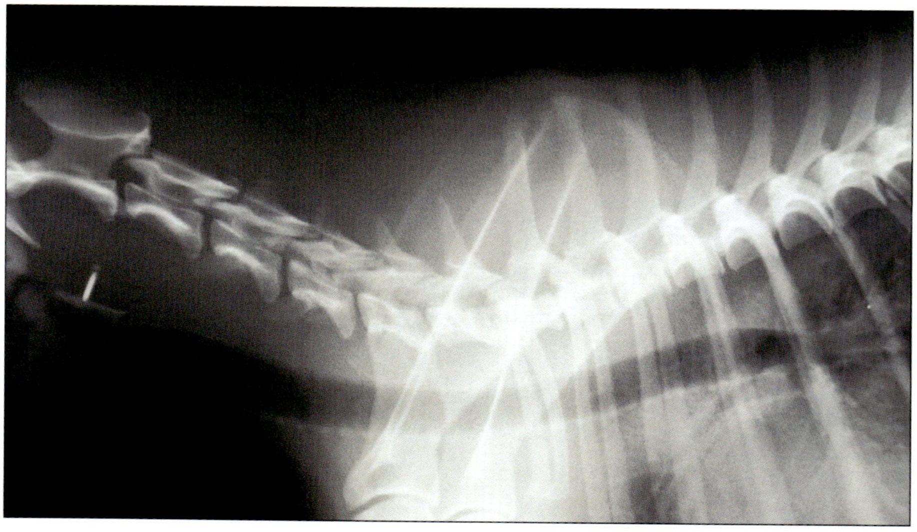

Fig. 3. Careless preparation will result in an image without diagnostic value.

After the lateral projection, a perpendicular image should be obtained: ventrodorsal (VD), or, in very special cases, dorsoventral (DV).

For the **ventrodorsal (VD)** projection (Figs. 4 and 5):

- Place the patient in dorsal recumbency.
- Ensure that there is no axial rotation with respect to the X-ray beam to avoid poor positioning that leads to an incorrect diagnosis. Foam wedges and sandbags placed either side of the thorax may be of assistance.
- Stretch the animal from the nose to the end of the column so that there is no iatrogenic deviation in any cervical segment.
- To obtain full extension and a good position of the vertebrae, a foam pad can be placed under the neck and a sandbag on the mandible.
- Pull both the forelimbs and the hind limbs caudally, if possible using positioning aids. In case of manual positioning, take adequate radio-protective measures and avoid the primary beam passing through the hands of the assistant. This should be the norm in any radiographic investigation.
- If the patient is under general anaesthesia and intubated, the endotracheal tube should be removed temporarily before taking the radiograph, as it may overlay the spine and interfere with the study.

For correct visualization of the cervical column in VD projection, the endotracheal tube should be removed if the patient is intubated.

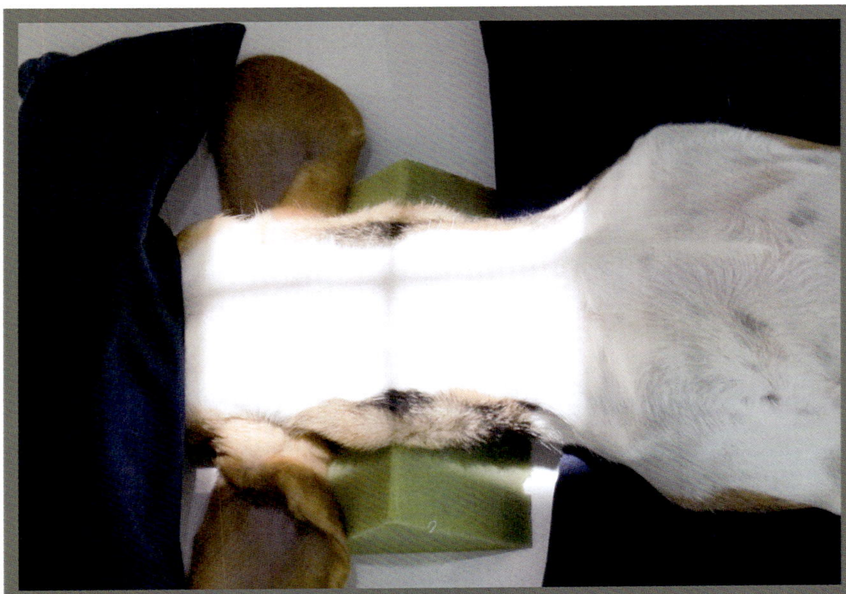

Fig. 4. Correct position for ventrodorsal projection of the cervical column.

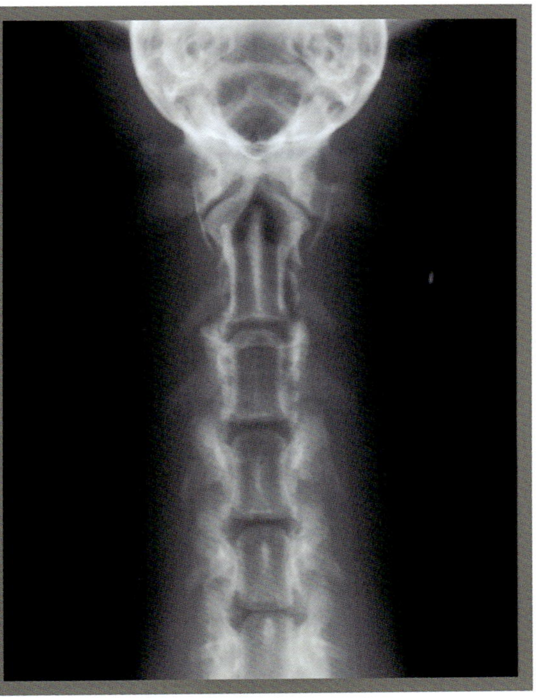

Fig. 5. VD radiograph of the cervical column. ▶

When **atlanto-axial subluxation** is suspected, a **rostrocaudal** or open-mouth projection may be added to the Lat projection (Figs. 6 and 7), using the following steps:

- Place the patient in dorsal recumbency.
- Flex the neck in such a way that the hard palate is at right angles to the radiographic cassette.
- Fix the mandible with adhesive tape and pull the tongue in a rostrocaudal direction with a soft tissue forceps.
- Centre the X-ray beam on the base of the tongue or on the soft palate.

This projection allows evaluation of the atlanto-axial joint, the shape and size of the foramen magnum and the presence or absence of the odontoid process and its shape and size. However, this is a **dangerous** projection if atlanto-axial subluxation is suspected, as it may exacerbate the clinical symptoms.

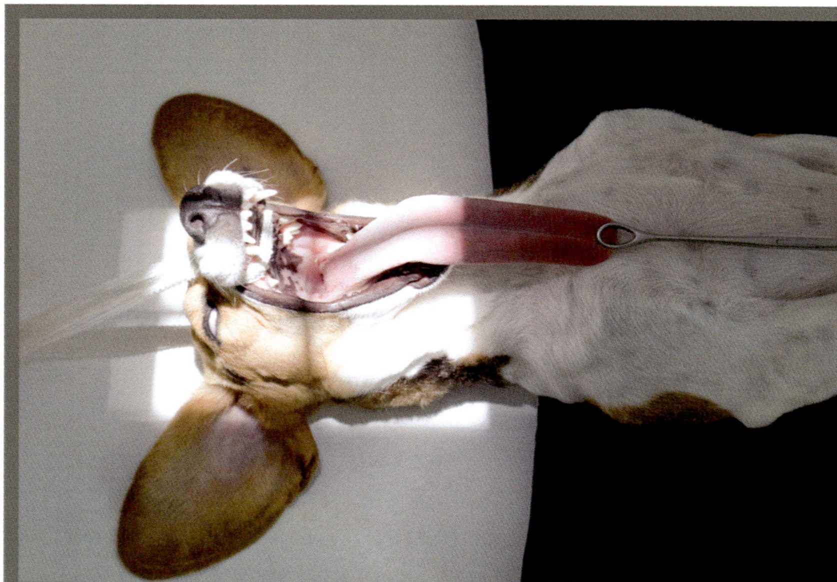

Fig. 6. Special open-mouth projection for atlanto-axial subluxation.

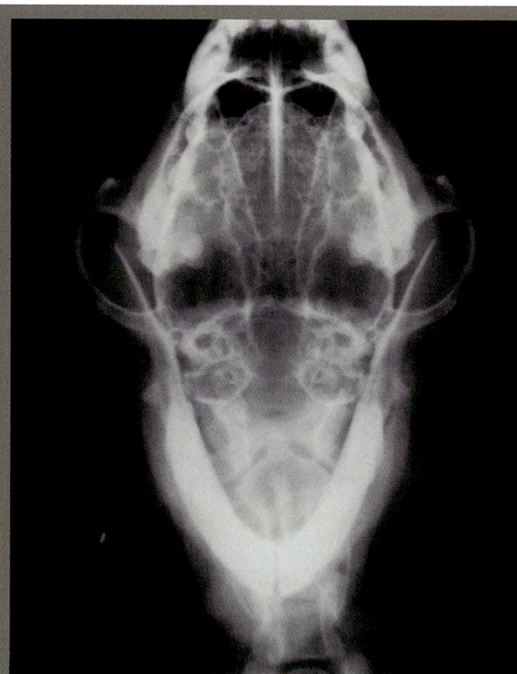

Fig. 7. Radiograph of the dog in figure 6. ▶

Thoracic column

Radiological examination of the thoracic column is used for the diagnosis of problems of the vertebrae (congenital malformations, fractures, dislocations, infections, neoplasia), the disc (herniation, infection) or the medulla (neoplasia).

It should be remembered at this point that, except in cases of severe spinal trauma, herniation of the disks of the vertebrae from T1 to T10 is highly unlikely, because the very strong capital ligament connecting the rib heads at this level makes it almost impossible for discs to protrude into the spinal canal.

For correct investigation of the full length of the thoracic column, it is usually necessary to take at least two radiographs in each of the basic projections, in this case the Lat and the VD.

> Due to its length, investigation of the thoracic column usually requires two radiographs each in VD and Lat projection.

For a correct **lateral (Lat)** projection (Figs. 8 and 9):

- Place the patient in lateral recumbency, with the forelimbs pulled out of the way cranially and the hind limbs caudally, and the limbs parallel to each other.
- Centre the X-ray beam on T8 if a lesion in the cranial thoracic column is suspected and on T13-L1 if a caudal lesion is suspected.
- Place a foam wedge under the sternum to avoid axial rotation, as the ventral thorax is usually narrower than the dorsal part. In this way, the X-ray beam is perfectly perpendicular to the thoracic vertebrae and superimposition of the rib heads on the vertebral canal is prevented, which is of particular importance if the latter is the structure being visualized.
- Collimate the X-ray beam as much as possible on the thoracic vertebrae, to avoid unnecessary scattered radiation. It should be remembered that when investigating the vertebral column, the rest of the thoracic structures should appear as little as possible on the radiograph.
- Although the patient should be in traction, the thoracic vertebrae are the least mobile of the whole spinal column, so that incomplete traction does not make a big difference to the end result.

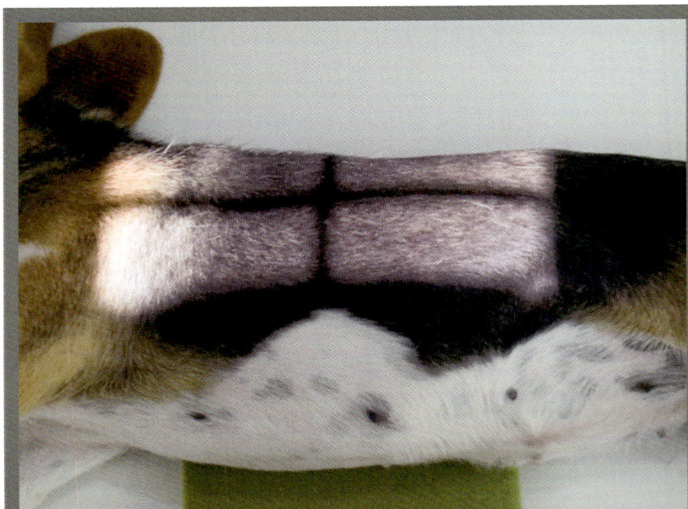

Fig. 8. Correct lateral position for investigation of the thoracic column.

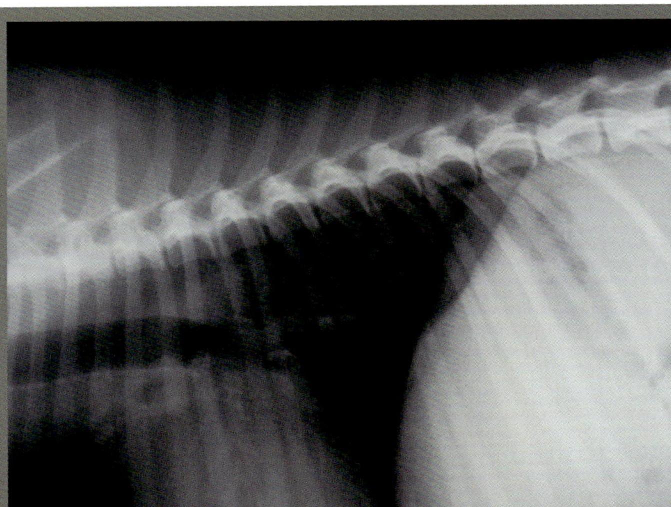

Fig. 9. Radiographic image of the thoracic column with a well-positioned patient.

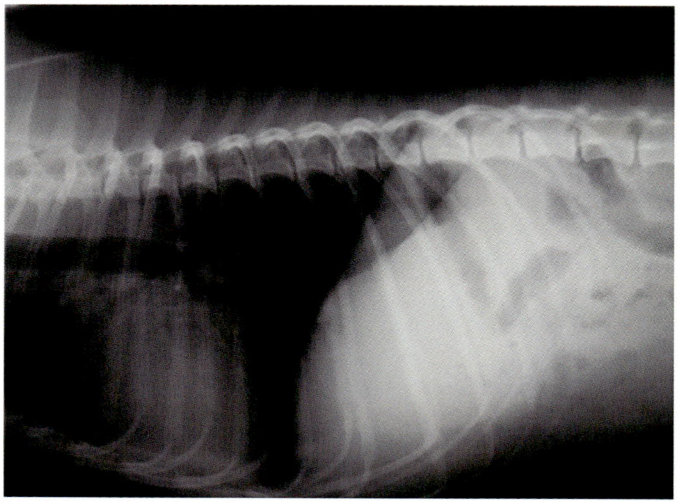

Fig. 10. If the X-ray beam is not perpendicular, diagnosis becomes difficult.

To avoid scattered radiation due to the thickness of the thorax, collimation of the X-ray beam should be tight when examining the thoracic column.

The most frequent mistake in this projection is an incorrect position of the foam wedge, as rotation with respect to the X-ray beam causes superimposition of the rib heads on the spinal canal (Fig. 10).

For the **ventrodorsal (VD)** projection (Figs. 11 and 12):

- Place the patient in dorsal recumbency, with the forelegs pulled forward and the hind legs backwards.
- Ensure that the X-ray beam is perfectly perpendicular to the area under examination. To obtain this, particularly in animals with a narrow thorax, a radiolucent cushion can be placed under the spinous processes, and sandbags on both sides to avoid rotation.
- A simple way to verify that the position is correct is to compare the length of the ribs on both sides. If they have the same length, the position is correct.

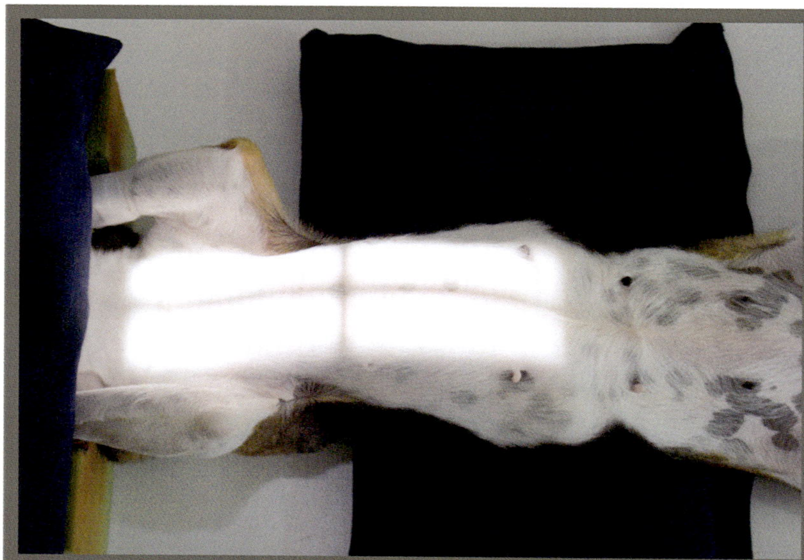

Fig. 11. Correct positioning for a good image of the thoracic column in ventrodorsal projection.

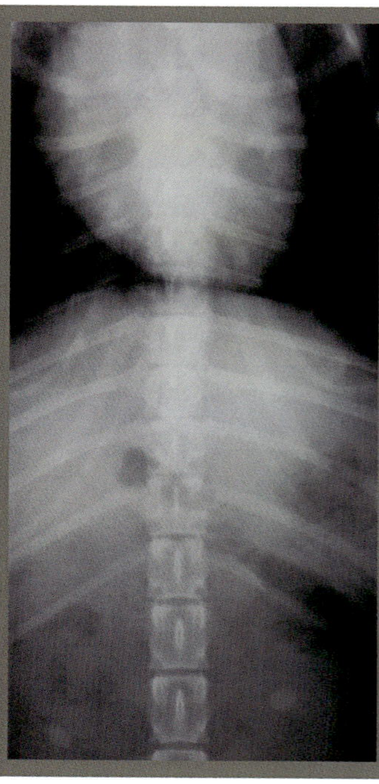

Fig. 12. Corresponding radiograph of the thoracic column in VD projection. ▶

Lumbar column

As with the cervical column, special care should be taken when examining the lumbar column, because this area is the most flexible of the whole spinal column after the cervical.

For a complete investigation, at least two perpendicular projections should be used, the lateral (Lat) and the ventrodorsal (VD), as the latter places the spinal column closer to the cassette, improving definition.

Starting with the **lateral (Lat)** projection (Figs. 13 and 14), one or two foam pads should be placed under the central lumbar vertebrae to compensate for the difference in height between the end of the thorax and the hip, and the central part of the lumbar column. This keeps the whole area parallel to the tabletop. The hind limbs should be pulled back, keeping them parallel to avoid rotation with respect to the beam. This can be achieved with a piece of rectangular foam between the stifles, so that the pelvis does not rotate.

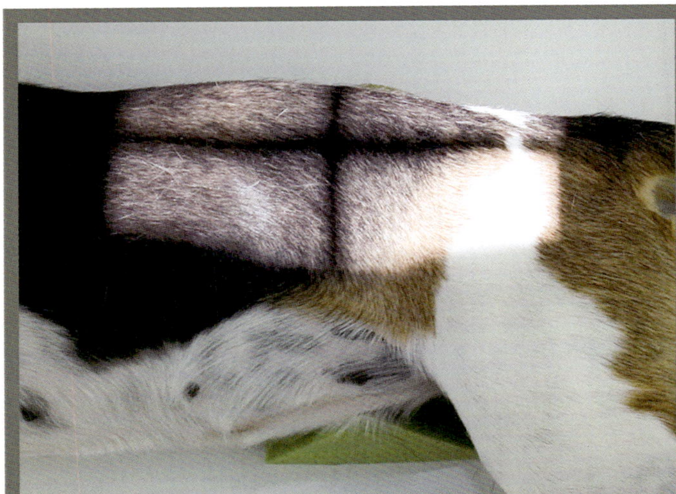

Fig. 13. Lateral projection of the lumbar column.

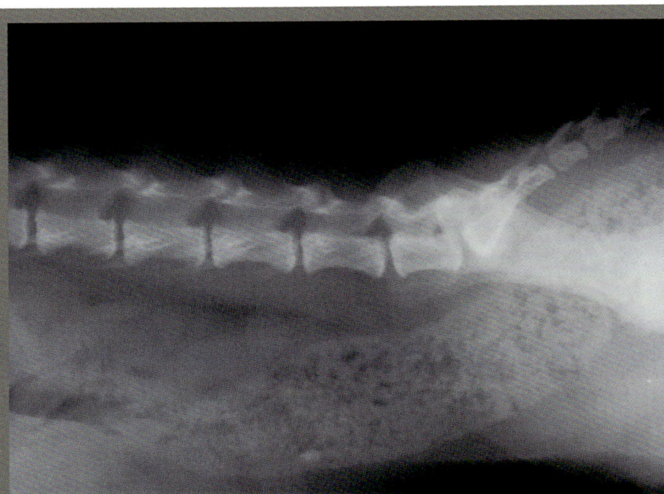

Fig. 14. Radiograph of a lateral projection of the lumbar column in a correct position.

In the lateral (Lat) projection the transverse processes should overlap, in such a way that each vertebra seems to have only one. When herniation of the disk is suspected, the **width of the intervertebral space** (a space that appears narrower between two wider ones) will indicate the probable location of the problem.

For the **ventrodorsal (VD)** projection (Figs. 15 and 16), the patient is placed in dorsal recumbency, with the forelimbs firmly stretched cranially and the hind limbs caudally; a relatively thin foam aid is placed under the lumbar vertebrae to avoid rotation with respect to the X-ray beam, especially if the animal has prominent spinous processes. Once again, the shape and size of the transverse processes are used to verify that the correct position has been achieved; they should be the same on both sides.

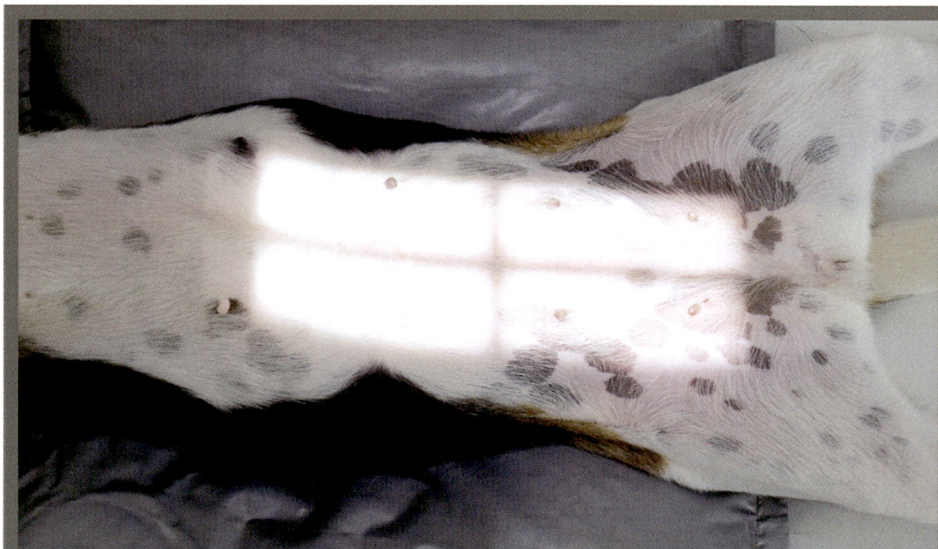

Fig. 15. Patient in the correct ventrodorsal position for investigation of the lumbar column.

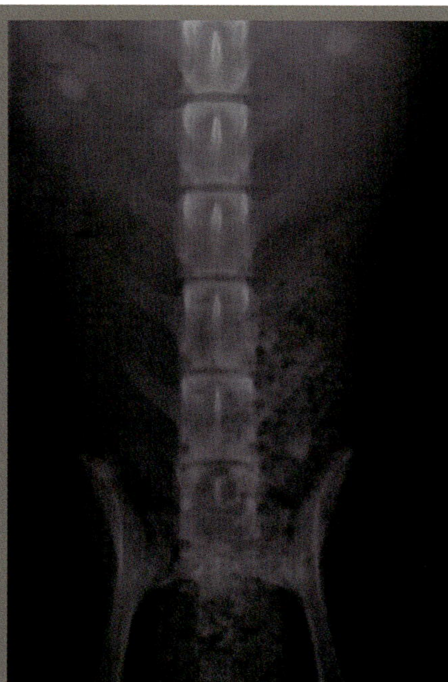

Fig. 16. With a good position, a good quality VD radiograph of the lumbar column is obtained. ▶

A rectangular piece of foam between the spinous processes and the table will help to avoid rotation.
An equal size of transverse processes on the radiograph is an indicator of correct positioning.

In cases of suspected herniation of a disc, this projection will not provide much information on the width of the intervertebral space. The projection requires special care when interpreting vertebral density, because of the superimposition of intestinal loops which, when full of gas, may lead to a mistaken suspicion of reduced density; which in turn may lead to erroneous diagnosis of an abnormality, such as a **vertebral neoplasia**. In male patients, a correct position means superimposition of the penile bone and the prepuce on the vertebrae, which sometimes makes interpretation difficult (Fig. 17).

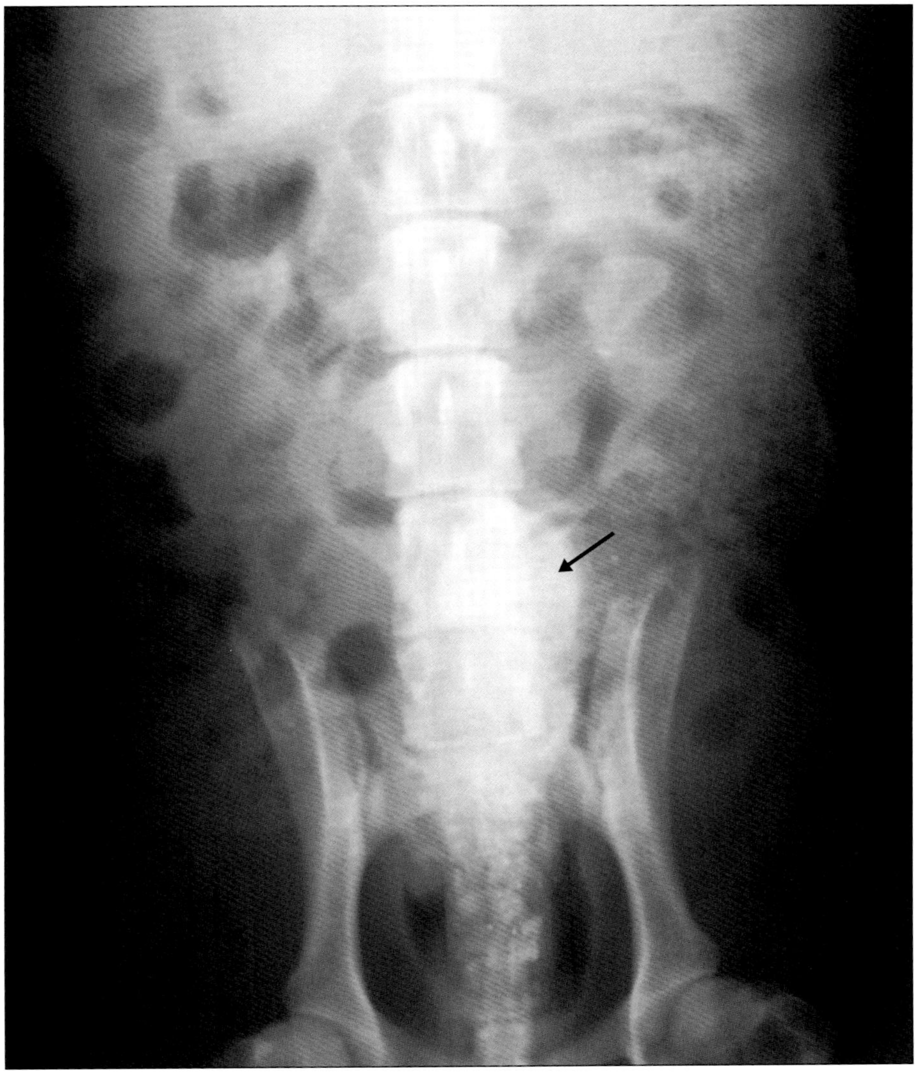

Fig. 17. In VD projection of the lumbar column, the penile bone and prepuce of male patients and the intestinal loops should be taken into account.

Lumbo-sacral column

For a complete investigation of the L7-S1 junction, the two usual perpendicular radiographs to be taken, are the **lateral (Lat)** and **ventrodorsal (VD)** projections.

The procedure for these positions is the same as for the lumbar column, that is, foam pieces should be placed under the central lumbar vertebrae and between the stifles in the Lat position, and under the last lumbar vertebrae and the sacrum in the VD position.

For the **Lat projection**, the hind limbs are pulled caudally without excessive force, such that L7 and S1 remain in a normal anatomical position as if the dog were standing. The ilial wings should appear in superimposition for a good assessment of the shape and size of the L7-S1 foramen and the width of the intervertebral space.

In **VD projection**, the position of the patient is identical to that for the lumbar column, but this time the X-ray beam is centred on the L7-S1 space.

When herniation of the disc is suspected in this area and myelography is performed, stress radiographs should be taken in two positions: forced flexion and extension.

In **forced flexion** (Figs. 18 and 19), the hind limbs are pulled forward between the forelegs and strong traction is applied, although always taking care that the legs remain parallel. Sometimes it is necessary to **increase the kV slightly** to obtain the same quality image as in standard Lat projection.

To obtain a good projection in **forced extension** (Figs. 20 and 21), the hind limbs are pulled caudally and a radiolucent aid (such as a bottle of alcohol) is used to press down the lumbar area in a ventral direction, which will put pressure on the area to be examined.

To obtain a good projection of the lumbo-sacral junction in forced extension, it is useful to press on the dorsum with a radiolucent object while at the same time applying traction to the hind legs.

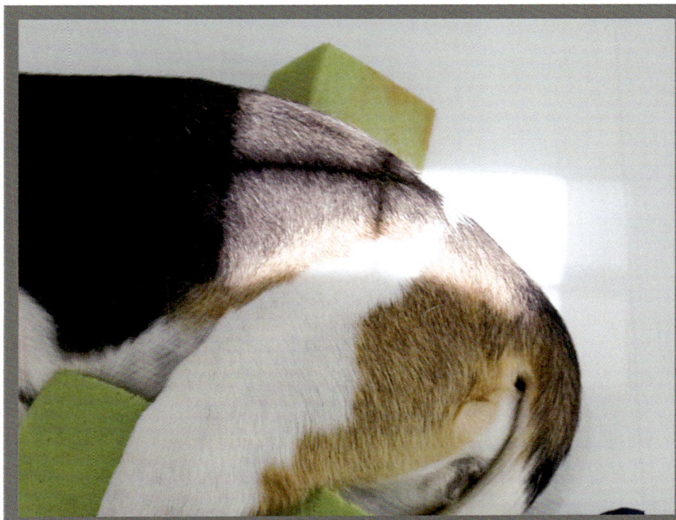

Fig. 18. Stress position of the lumbo-sacral column in forced flexion.

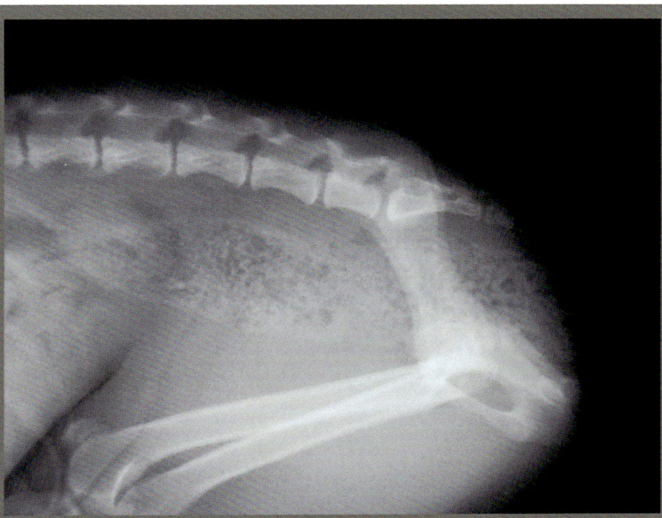

Fig. 19. Radiological projection of the picture on the left.

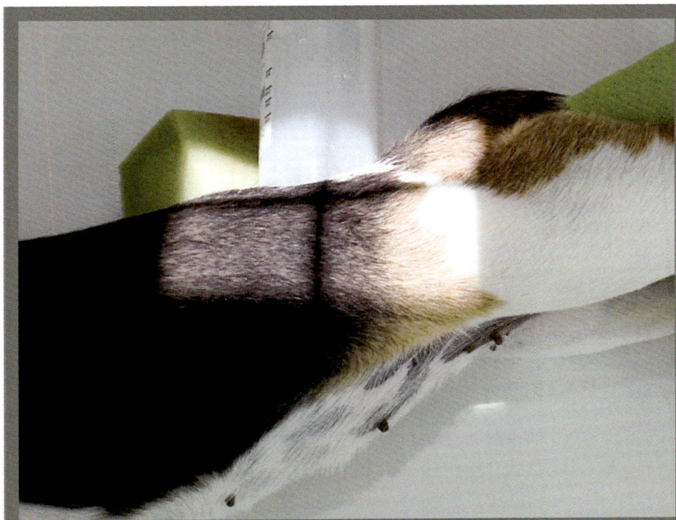

Fig. 20. Stress position of the lumbo-sacral column in forced extension.

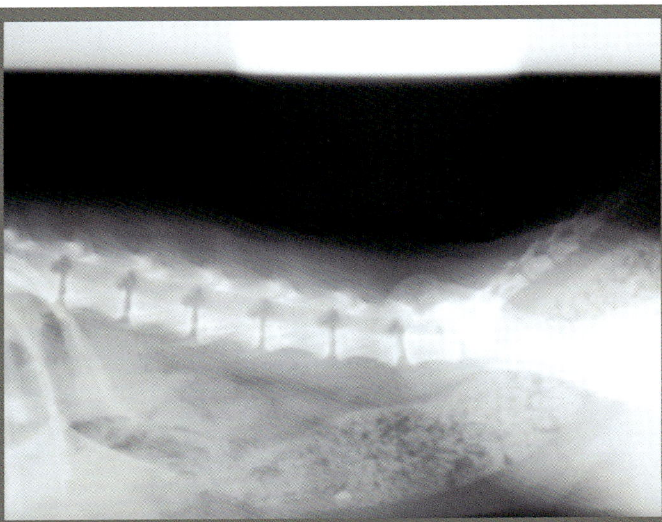

Fig. 21. Corresponding radiograph of the lumbo-sacral column in forced extension.

Myelography

This technique is used for radiographic examination of the spinal cord and consists of the introduction of a positive contrast medium into the subarachnoid space to visualize the medullary outline. Before performing myelography, the clinical history of the patient and two plain radiographs in Lat and VD position should be available.

Indications

- Exact location of herniated discs.
- Traumatic lesions of the vertebrae.
- Medullary lesions.
- When basic radiology does not concur with neurological assessment.

Contraindications

- When general anaesthesia is contraindicated (shock, uraemia, etc.).
- If plain radiography provides an exact diagnosis (rare).
- If analysis of the cerebrospinal fluid indicates infection, in which case the symptoms may be exacerbated.
- If neurological assessment determines the nature and location of the lesion.

Technique

- Premedication: it is better not to use phenothiazines, as they lower the threshold for convulsions. A diazepam-atropine combination can be used.
- Preparation of puncture site, shave and disinfect.
- Anaesthesia with sodium thiopental or propofol.
- Endotracheal intubation, halothane or isofluorane and oxygen.
- Contrast medium: iohexol, non-ionic, water-soluble, at a concentration of 240, 270 or 300 mg/ml.

Cervical myelography

The puncture is performed in the cisterna magna. The animal is placed in right lateral recumbency, although sternal recumbency can be used too. The sagittal plane should be parallel to the tabletop and the neck is flexed until the tip of the nose is at a right angle. (Fig. 22).

At this point, it is very important to deflate the cuff of the endotracheal tube to avoid collapse, unless it is kink resistant (internal reinforcing wire spiral). Use 20 to 23 G spinal needles with a length of 40 to 70 mm, depending on the size of the patient.

A thumb is placed on the central area of the wing of the atlas and the middle finger on the external occipital crest. The puncture is performed exactly in the midline and halfway between the wing and the crest, with the bevel directed caudally to avoid contrast medium flowing towards the cerebral ventricles. The needle is pushed in slowly and when the ligamenta flava and dura mater are perforated, there is a characteristic pop and resistance decreases. Although the books say that this is the moment to withdraw the stylet, the authors withdraw it just before they believe they are reaching the subarachnoid space, because that way the flow of cerebrospinal fluid indicates that the space has been reached. The first drops may be slightly blood-stained because of muscle perforation, but the procedure may be continued if, after waiting a few moments, the fluid becomes clear. If the fluid turns out to be blood, the needle should be withdrawn and another needle should be used. If this happens 2 or 3 times, it is better to try a lumbar puncture or repeat the procedure at a different time. The amount of fluid that flows out should be approximately the same as the volume of contrast injected. Fluid should never be extracted with a syringe, as this may provoke a cerebellar hernia, which would be extremely serious.

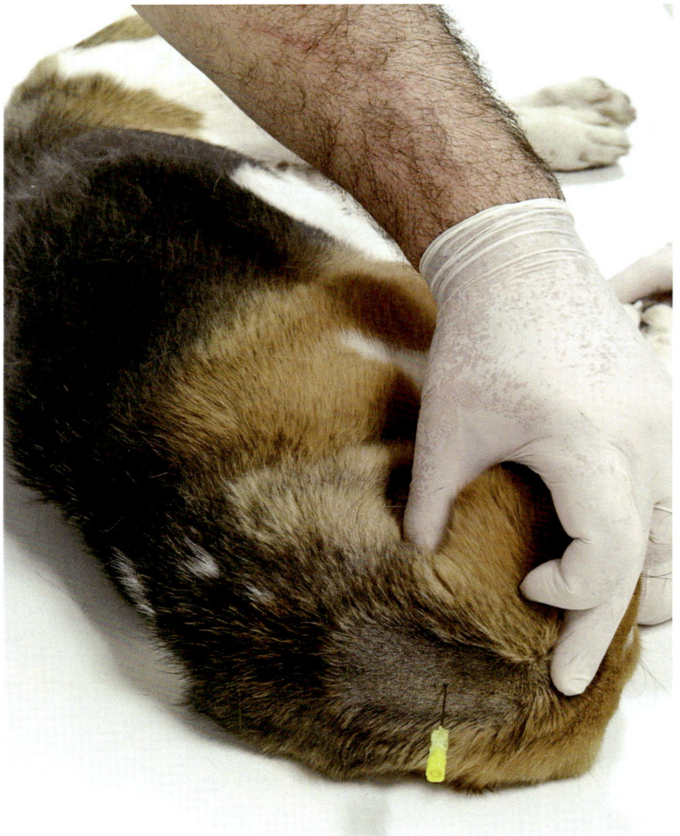

Fig. 22. Correct position for a cervical puncture.

It is advisable to raise the animal's head to avoid contrast filling the cerebral ventricles.

> When performing a cervical puncture for myelography, it is advisable to raise the head from the table as soon as the spinal needle is withdrawn, to prevent contrast medium flowing toward the cerebral ventricles.

Lumbar myelography

This technique is safer in principle, but is also more difficult to perform, in particular in obese or very big animals, and the results are not always as expected. In general, it is used for cases of thoraco-lumbar or lumbar intervertebral disc disease, or for cats or very small dogs. The patient is placed in lateral or sternal recumbency; the authors prefer right lateral recumbency with the hind limbs pulled forward taking care to keep the spine completely parallel to the table (Fig. 23).

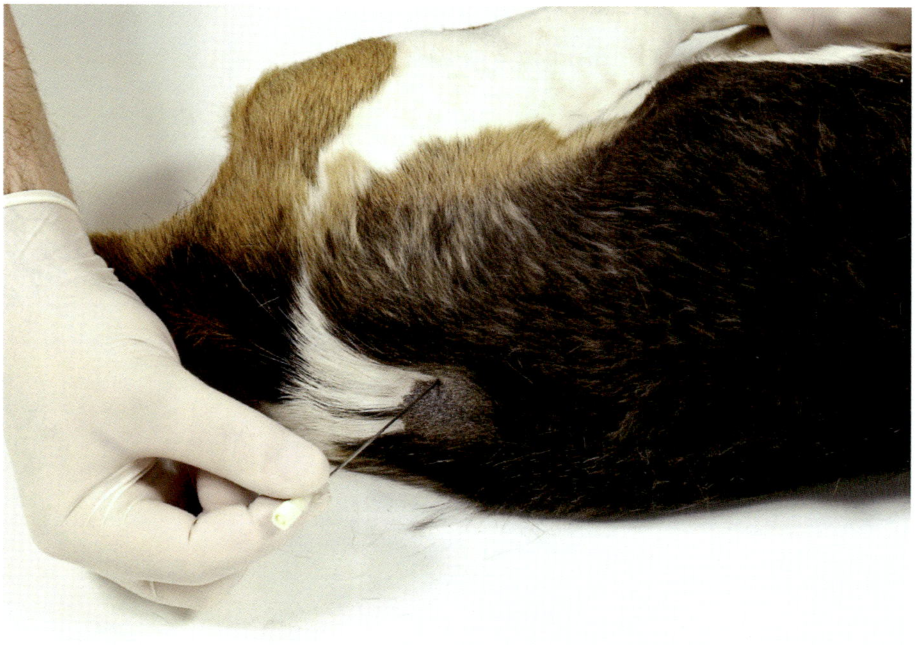

Fig. 23. Position for lumbar puncture in right lateral recumbency.

The area is prepared in the same way and the puncture can be performed between L4 and L5 or L5 and L6. If the latter is chosen, the caudal part of the spinous process of L6 is identified; which is normally the first that can be palpated cranial to the wings of the ilium. The needle is inserted slightly off the midline and pushed in a cranioventral direction at an angle of 30 to 60°, just lateral to the spinous process (it is best to keep very close to the process until hitting the dorsal arch and then direct the needle cranially until the space between the arches is found). In older animals or large breeds, this procedure sometimes has to be repeated several times until the subarachnoid space is reached, because of dorsal osteophytes in the midline.

When the needle perforates the dura mater, the tail and hind limbs may suffer an involuntary contraction, which has no pathological significance.

Usually, the needle is inserted to the bottom of the medullary canal, then slowly withdrawn, and with the bevel in cranial direction the stylet is removed and the cerebrospinal fluid should start to flow. In cats or small dogs this is usually the case, but in big dogs, the needle should sometimes be withdrawn slightly for this to happen. If nothing happens, the correct position of the needle should be verified by fluoroscopy or radiography.

For lumbar puncture, cross the medulla until reaching the bottom of the canal, then withdraw the needle slightly and wait for the fluid to flow when the stylet is removed.

The contrast medium can be injected through an extension tube rather than connecting the syringe straight to the needle, which will avoid displacement of the needle towards the epidural space or medulla. The radiological images that will be obtained if the projections are correct can be seen in figures 24 to 26.

Complications

- Due to general anaesthesia.
- Due to the puncture technique.
- Convulsions: different authors describe their occurrence in 15 to 40% of cases, although in the authors' experience this percentage is 5% or less, because they use iohexol which is very safe. It is advisable to maintain anaesthesia for 30 minutes after finishing the procedure and if convulsions start, administer intravenous diazepam at a dose rate of 10-20 mg and a corticosteroid.

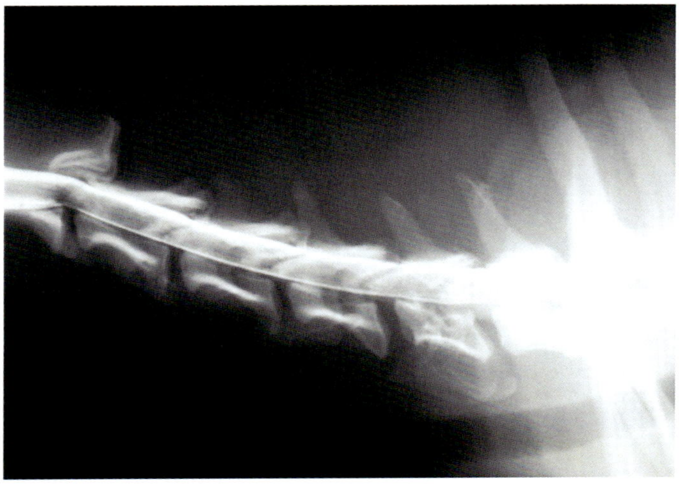

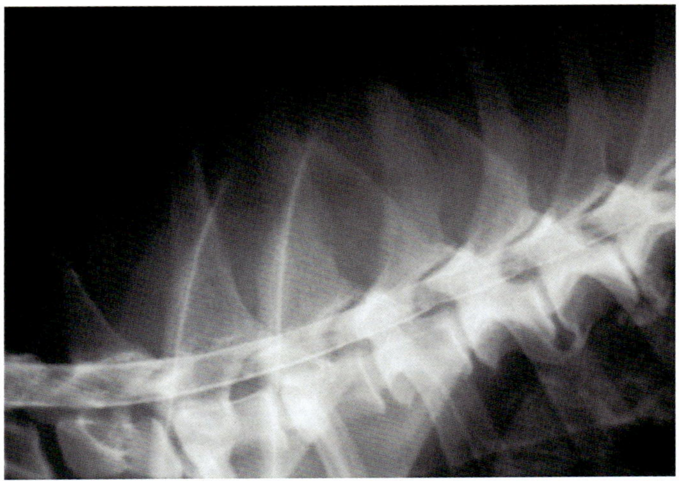

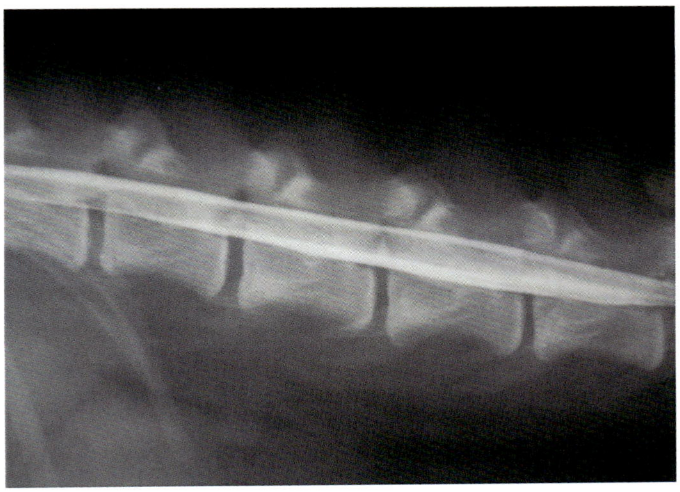

Figs. 24, 25 and 26. In a healthy animal, the contrast medium fills the whole subarachnoid space and generally reaches the lumbo-sacral area after 10-15 minutes.

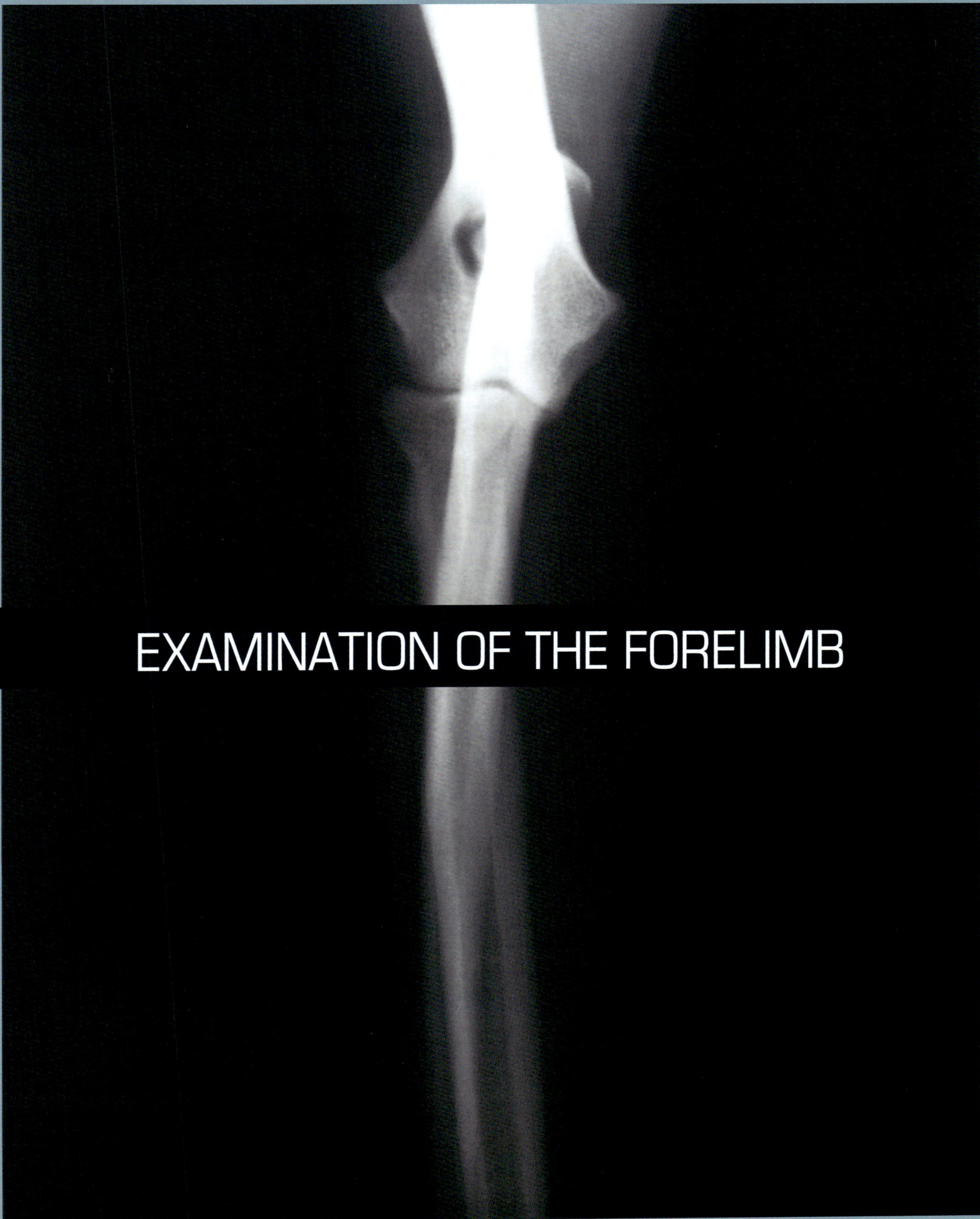

EXAMINATION OF THE FORELIMB

General considerations

For radiological examination of the forelimb, it is usually sufficient to sedate the patient, except in case of very painful fractures or dislocations, when deep sedation or general anaesthesia should be used to allow better diagnostic positioning of the area concerned.

As a general rule, the X-ray beam should be collimated as much as possible to minimize scattered radiation that will degrade the image; it also affects the attending staff, if any, although their presence during exposure should be avoided if possible.

Again, with the aim to reduce scattered radiation on the image to a minimum, an anti-scatter grid should be used if the structure to be radiographed is thicker than 10-15 cm. In general, the structures of the forelimb above the elbow joint require its use, with the possible exception of small dogs, in which the thickness is practically always less than 10 cm. For examination of the elbow itself or the structures below it, a grid may be unnecessary and the cassette is placed directly on the X-ray table.

Exposure factors

To examine the appendicular skeleton, generally **the kilovoltage should not be too high**, between 45 and 70 kV depending on the area, and the **milliamperage-second (mAs) should be relatively high**, although its setting depends on the type of film and whether a grid is used (it should always be higher with a grid).

If there is clinical suspicion of neoplasia or infection, a cassette with the screen and film used for mammography is very useful. The definition of the image will be much improved, so that it is possible to spot details that would otherwise go unnoticed. The disadvantage of mammography film is that it requires an important increase in mAs (up to 5 times).

Generally, a low kV and a relatively high mAs are used for radiological examination of the appendicular skeleton, depending on the film.

Even though the mineral content of the appendicular skeleton provides good radiological contrast, it should be remembered that other structures with soft tissue radiopacity, such as peri-articular or intra-articular areas, should also be visualized on the radiograph, which is why **overexposure of the image should always be avoided**.

The different projections for examination of each structure of the forelimb will be discussed by area, but in general, anterioposterior (AP) projections will need a 10% increase in kilovoltage as compared to mediolateral (ML) projections, because the tissues in AP projection are thicker.

During radiological examination of the appendicular skeleton, overexposure should be avoided, in order to visualize the peri-articular and intra-articular soft tissues.

Positions and projections

In general, examination of all the structures of the forelimb requires at least two perpendicular projections, most commonly the mediolateral (ML) and the anteroposterior (AP) or posteroanterior (PA). The latter are called craniocaudal (CrCd) or caudocranial (CdCr) when referring to structures above the carpus, and dorsopalmar/palmodorsal when referring to the carpus or below. Apart from the above projections, other special projections will be described in this chapter.

Hereafter, each area will be discussed, starting at the proximal end of the limb and finishing with the phalanges.

Scapula

For radiological examination of the scapula, the mediolateral (ML) and caudocranial (CdCr) projections are used.

As discussed previously, if the area to be radiographed is thicker than 10 cm, an anti-scatter grid should be used.

In **mediolateral (ML)** projection, the difficulty is that a large area of the scapula overlies the thorax and the spinal column. Therefore, it is necessary to choose whether to focus on the distal part of the scapular body, the neck and the glenoid cavity, or the proximal part of the body and the spine of the scapula, because the projections employed are different, as will be discussed.

For examination of the scapula, it should be decided beforehand on which part to focus on, as the superimposition of several structures makes this a complex area.

For examination of the **distal end of the scapular body, the neck and the glenoid cavity:**

- Place the patient in lateral recumbency, with the affected side on the table.
- The affected limb should be pulled cranially, avoiding rotation, while the other limb should be pulled caudally to avoid superimposition, flexing the elbow slightly.
- The primary beam should be centred on the neck of the scapula (Fig. 1).

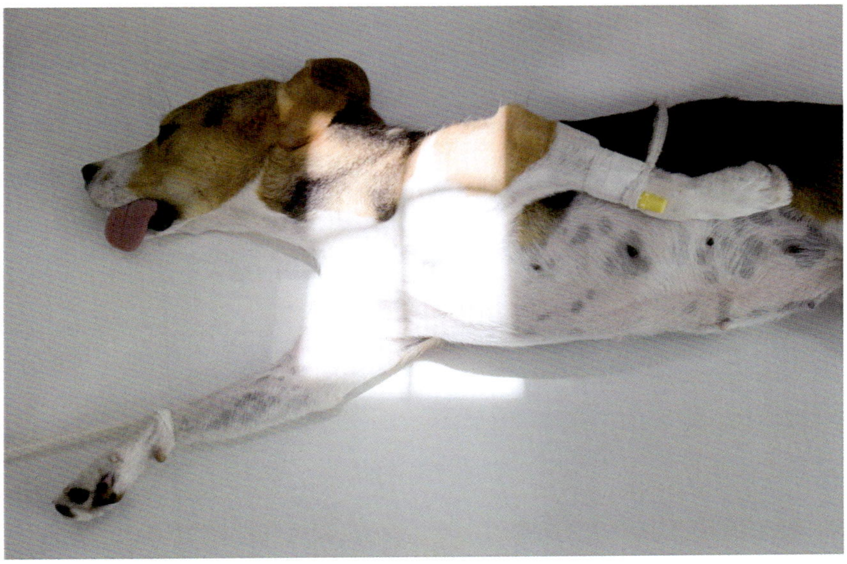

Fig. 1. Correct position for examination of the distal scapula in mediolateral projection.

For the **proximal scapular body and spine**:

- Place the patient on the table on its healthy side.
- Pull the affected limb caudally and the healthy limb cranially, i.e. the opposite of the previous projection. In this way, the affected scapula will contrast with the air in the lungs and will be easier to visualize.
- The primary beam should be centred on the middle third of the scapular body.

The **caudocranial (CdCr)** projection is more useful than the craniocaudal projection and also makes positioning much easier. For this projection:

- Place the patient in dorsal recumbency, with the affected limb in forced traction in a cranial direction, in such a way that the scapula is as parallel as possible to the table (Fig. 2).
- Avoid external rotation of the limb, as this may make interpretation difficult.
- It is useful to rotate the body slightly towards the healthy side to align the affected limb. The healthy limb can be tied back or left loose with a weight on the axillary area, to avoid rotation of the body.
- The X-ray beam should be centred on the central part of the scapula.

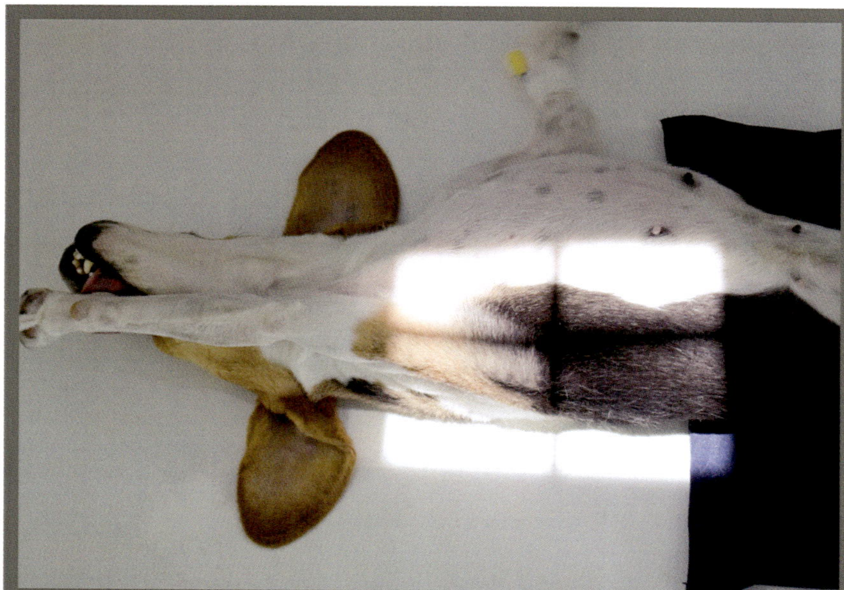

Fig. 2. Patient in position for caudocranial examination of the scapula.

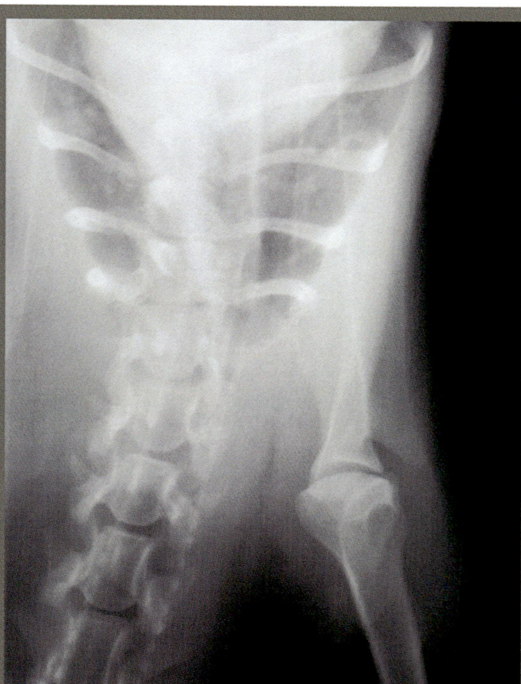

Fig. 3. Radiograph of the scapula in CdCr projection. ▶

Shoulder

Routine radiological examination of the shoulder requires mediolateral and caudocranial projections. An additional skyline projection may be carried out to detect lesions of the tendons or muscles.

For a good **mediolateral (ML)** projection of the shoulder joint, the position of the patient is similar to the one for examination of the distal scapula. That is:

- The patient is placed in lateral recumbency, with the affected limb against the table, under cranial traction.
- The other forelimb should be pulled back caudally to avoid superimposition, but without excessive force, as this might cause rotation of the affected joint and lead to a diagnostic error, in particular when looking for dislocation or subluxation of the joint (Figs. 4 and 5).

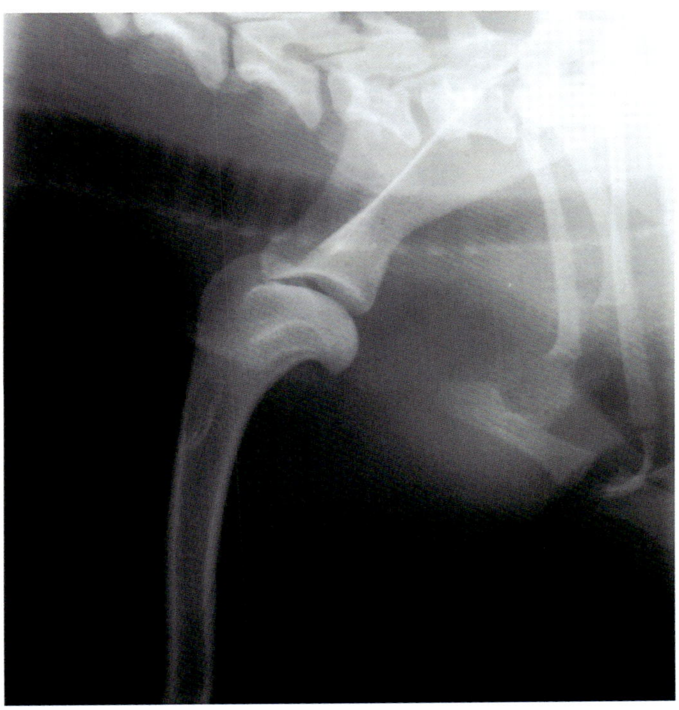

Fig. 4. Radiograph of the shoulder in a correct position to assess the joint cavity in ML projection.

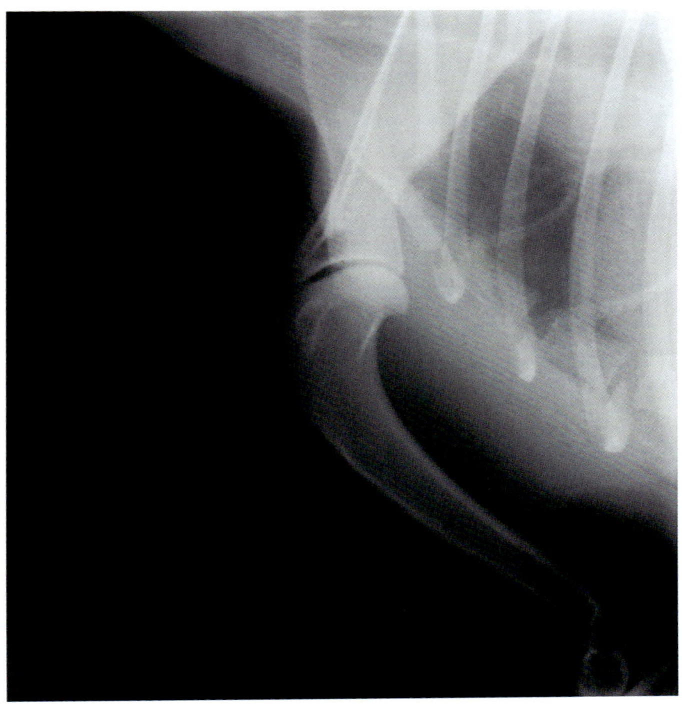

Fig. 5. Radiograph of a poorly-positioned shoulder in ML projection.

- The head and neck should be gently extended in dorsal direction to avoid superimposition of the trachea on the shoulder joint.
- The anatomical reference for the central beam is the scapular acromion (Fig. 6).

To examine the shoulder, the CdCr projection provides more information than the CrCd and is also easier to perform, although it requires deep sedation or general anaesthesia.

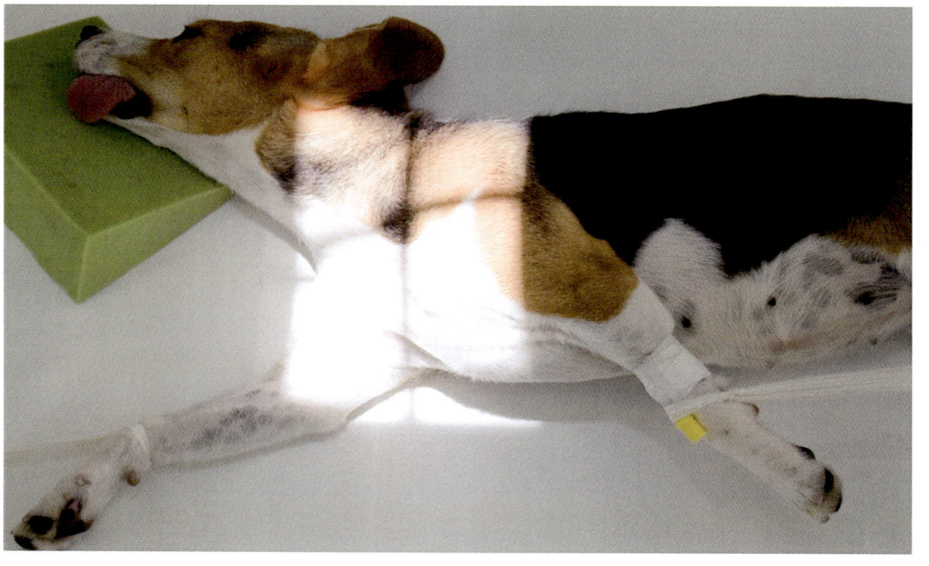

Fig. 6. The beam should be centred on the acromion in mediolateral projection.

The **caudocranial** (CdCr) projection is the most suitable for examination of the shoulder joint, as the craniocaudal projection is almost impossible to carry out and thus rarely turns out well-positioned. In general, and in particular if there is suspicion of a severe lesion, the animal should be at least sedated and often anaesthetised. Positioning:

- Place the patient in dorsal recumbency with the affected limb in firm traction in a cranial direction (Fig. 7).
- The other forelimb should be pulled back caudally, trying to keep the two limbs parallel, so as to maintain the body in this position. A rigid wedge under the caudal part of the thorax is useful to maintain this position.
- Turn the body slightly towards the healthy limb, as this manoeuvre tends to improve the alignment between the scapula and the humerus, which is helpful in cases of suspected subluxation of the shoulder. If this is not done, or if the joint is rotated the other way towards the affected side, an incorrect diagnosis of instability may be reached, because the middle part of the joint cavity tends to appear widened, but this is not pathological.
- The primary beam should be centred once more on the scapular acromion.

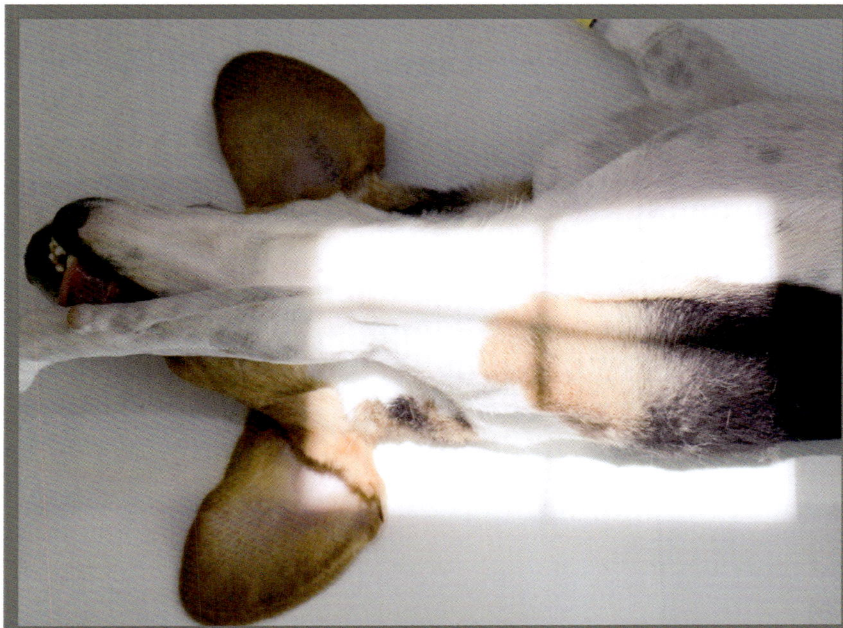

Fig. 7. Correct position of the patient for caudocranial projection of the shoulder.

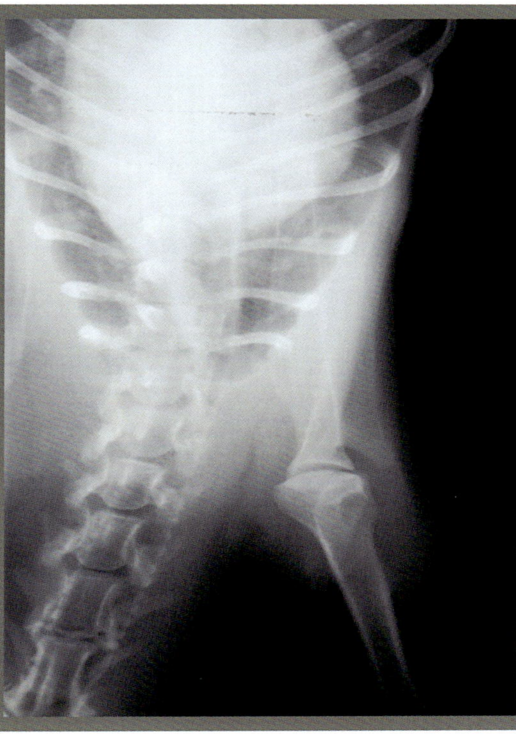

Fig. 8. Radiological image of the shoulder in CdCr projection. ▶

The **tangential (skyline)** projection is an additional projection for the shoulder joint.

This is a special projection for which both the shoulder and the elbow should be brought into maximum flexion, which means that the patient has to be deeply sedated or anaesthetised, because this is very difficult to achieve in a conscious patient. This projection allows visualization of the groove through which the tendon of the biceps brachii muscle runs and of the insertion area of the supraspinatus and infraspinatus muscles, when looking for mineralisation in any of these tendons. For the tangential projection (Fig. 9):

- Place the animal in sternal recumbency. With foam positioning aids, the head and healthy limb are raised and the healthy limb is flexed to support the body and avoid rotation. The head may also be turned towards the healthy side to avoid interference with the image.
- Both the shoulder and the elbow of the affected limb must be maintained in maximum flexion, while keeping them parallel to the body so as to obtain a diagnostic position.
- The X-ray beam is centred on the intertubercular groove of the humerus and care should be taken that the foot and carpus of the patient are moved out of the way to avoid superimposition.
- As the X-ray beam must be collimated maximally in this type of projection, the cassette is placed directly on the table. The image obtained can be seen in figure 10.

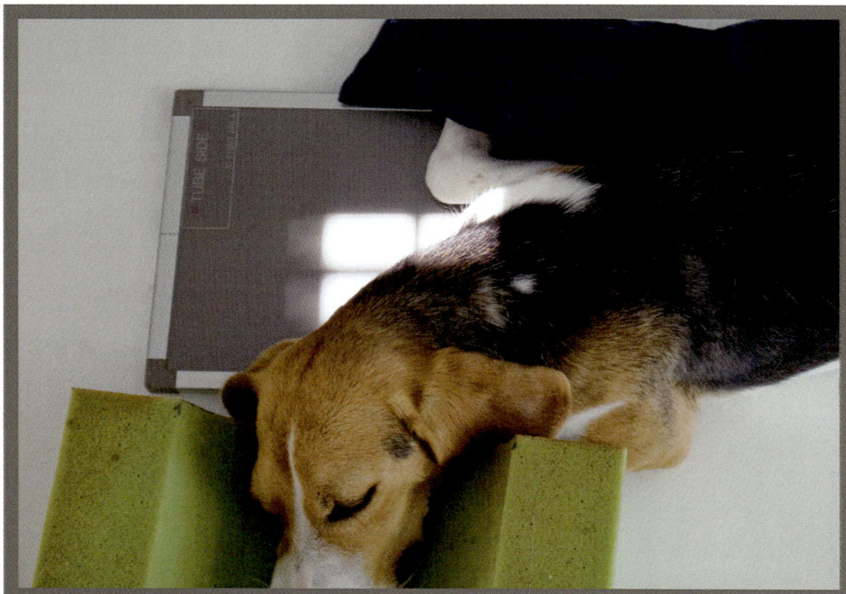

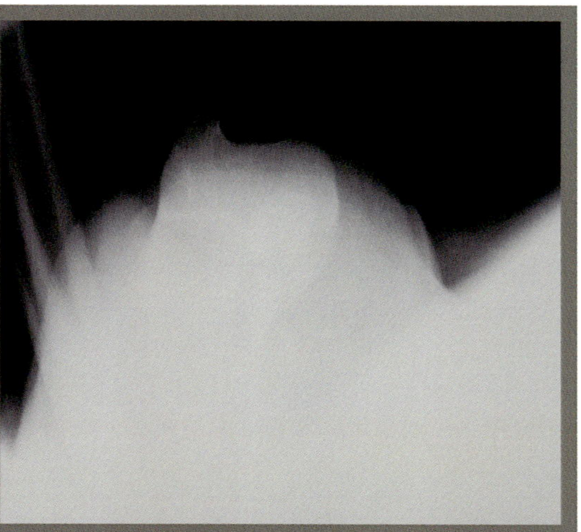

Fig. 10. Radiograph obtained with skyline projection.

Fig. 9. Skyline projection of the shoulder requires a special position of the patient.

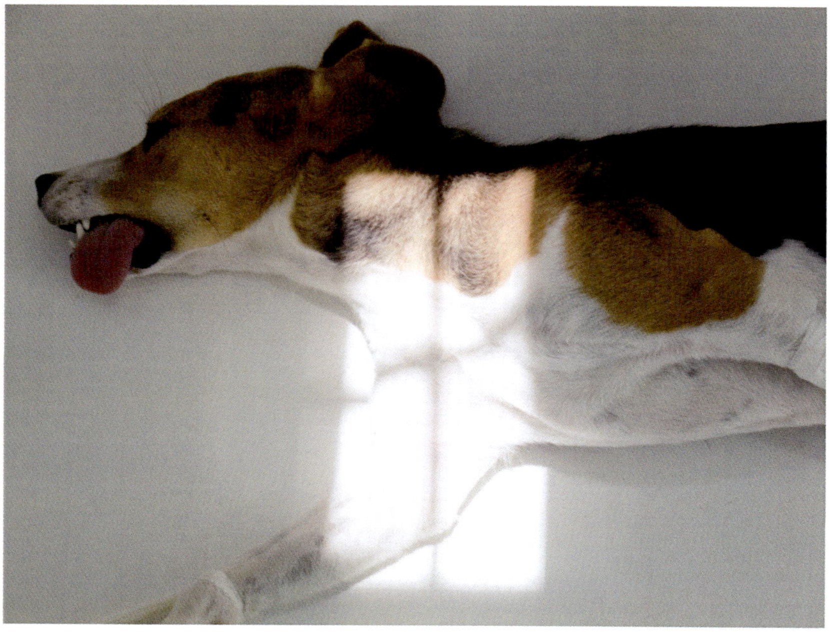

Fig. 11. The beam is centred at the midpoint of the humeral diaphysis.

Humerus

For radiological examination of the humerus the mediolateral and caudocranial projections are used.

For **mediolateral (ML)** projection of the humerus:

- Place the patient in lateral recumbency with the affected side on the table.
- The affected limb is pulled cranially and the healthy limb caudally, without excessive force, because otherwise the affected humerus lifts up from the table and ceases to be parallel to the cassette, which will distort the image.
- The neck and head are moved out of the way dorsally.
- In this case, the primary beam is centred on the humeral diaphysis (Fig. 11).

For **caudocranial (CdCr)** projection:

- Place the patient in dorsal recumbency and maintain this position with a foam wedge against the back and a weight on the healthy limb.
- Pull the affected limb cranially, applying firm traction to situate the humerus as parallel as possible to the table.
- Avoid rotation of the limb by turning the body slightly towards the healthy side.
- Direct the central beam on the midpoint of the diaphysis.

This position is much more frequently used than the craniocaudal position, as it allows for much more realistic visualization of the complete humeral anatomy. **Cranio-caudal (CrCd)** projection is only used in cases of serious fractures of the humerus or elbow joint, which do not permit much traction. For this projection, the affected limb is pulled caudally, close to the body, and the body is rotated slightly towards it to avoid superimposition with the ribs (Fig. 12).

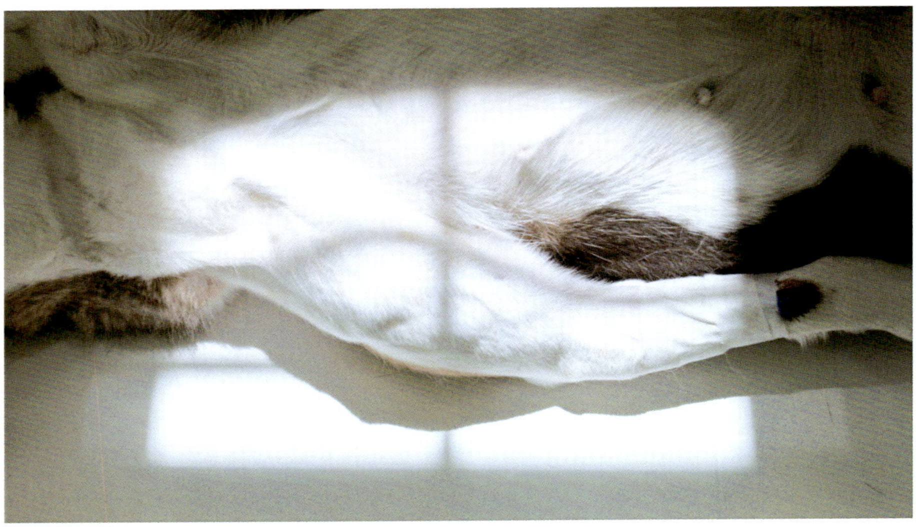

Fig. 12. For craniocaudal projection, the body is rotated slightly towards the affected side.

The craniocaudal projection for examination of the humeral anatomy is only used in cases of serious fractures, which do not permit much traction.

Elbow

For radiological examination of the elbow, with its complex anatomical structure, different projections can be used that make it possible to assess the complete joint.

As discussed in the general considerations, from the elbow down it is rarely necessary to use an anti-scatter grid, because, as long as the beam is sufficiently collimated, the amount of scattered radiation will be minimal due to the reduced thickness of the area.

First, the **mediolateral (ML)** projection is described, which is always the first option in any radiological study of the elbow. For this projection:

- Place the patient in lateral recumbency with the affected side on the table (Fig. 13).
- Pull the affected limb cranially.
- Pull the healthy limb caudally and secure it there.
- Centre the primary beam on the medial epicondyle of the humerus.
- Move the head and neck slightly dorsally out of the way.

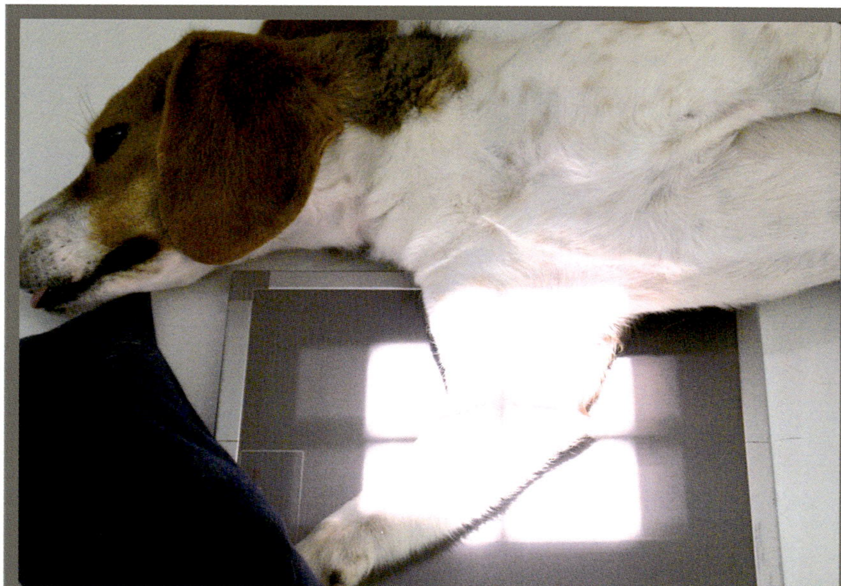

Fig. 13. This is the position for an image of the elbow in mediolateral projection.

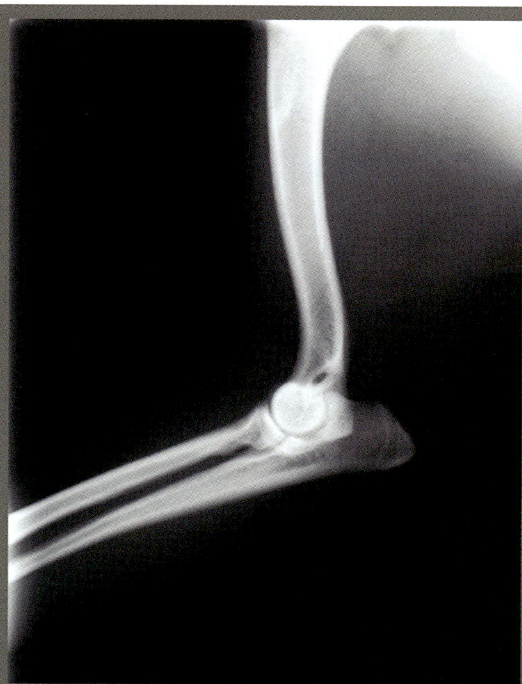

Fig. 14. Radiograph of the elbow in ML projection. ▶

With this projection (Fig. 14), an excellent assessment of **joint congruity** is possible, when dysplasia of the elbow is suspected.

Another projection used for the elbow joint is the **neutral ML**, in which everything is identical to the previous position, except that in this case the elbow is flexed by approximately 90°. This may useful for **visualization of fractures** and to assess **the state of the subchondral bone caudal to the semilunar notch of the ulna**.

Occasionally, in particular when elbow dysplasia is suspected, a **ML projection in forced flexion** is required (Fig. 15). This is already required by certain breed societies. The position of the animal is the same as for the two previous projections, but this time the radiograph is taken with the elbow in maximal flexion, in order to avoid superimposition of the anconeal process of the ulna on the epicondyles of the humerus. In this way, its dorsal surface can be checked for osteophytes and the separation of the anconeal process from the ulna in case of **ununited anconeal process** can be assessed.

To avoid rotation of the elbow in this position, a foam wedge is placed under the foot and carpus.

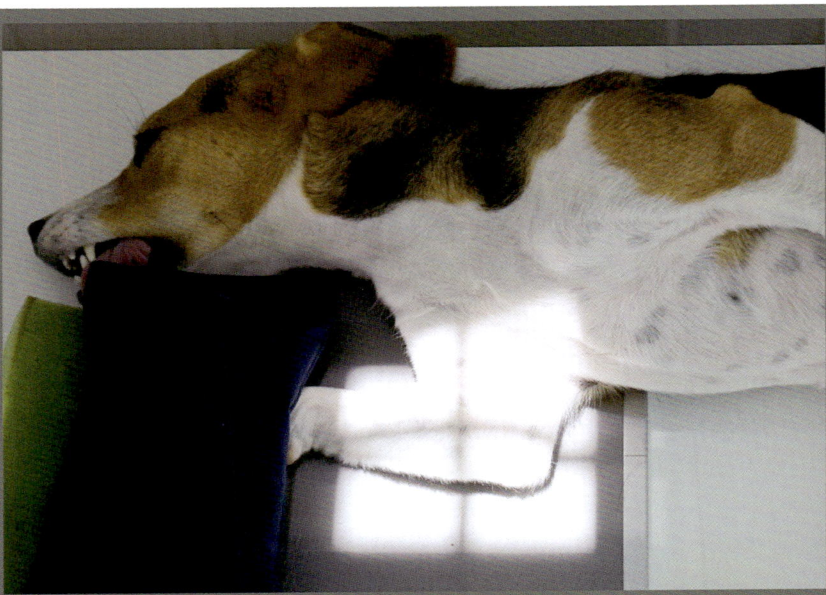

Fig. 15. Correct position for examination of the elbow in mediolateral projection with forced flexion.

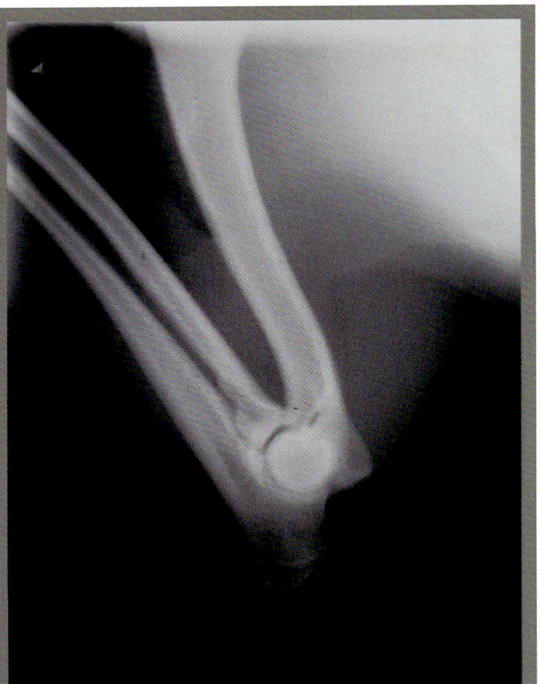

Fig. 16. Radiograph of the elbow in ML projection with forced flexion. ▶

The projection of the elbow in forced flexion allows correct visualization of the whole anconeal process of the ulna, as there is no superimposition on the humeral epicondyles.

Another projection that is used is the **caudocranial (CdCr)** projection, for which it is usually necessary to sedate or anaesthetise the animal, because traction is often painful. This projection is very useful for assessing the presence of osteophytes in the area of the **medial coronoid process of the ulna**, when suspecting its fragmentation. For this projection:

- Place the patient in dorsal recumbency, with the healthy limb held down on the table by a weight, such as a sandbag, or maintaining the position with a foam wedge against the back.
- Apply firm traction to the affected limb in a cranial direction and tie it there, trying to bring the elbow as close as possible to the X-ray table.
- Avoid rotation of the joint by turning the body slightly towards the healthy limb.
- Centre the primary beam on the distal end of the humerus (Fig. 17).

This is also the best projection when suspecting **osteochondrosis or OCD of the medial condyle of the humerus**, as the X-rays cross the surface of the joint parallel to the joint surface, which provides the best possible visualization (Fig. 18).

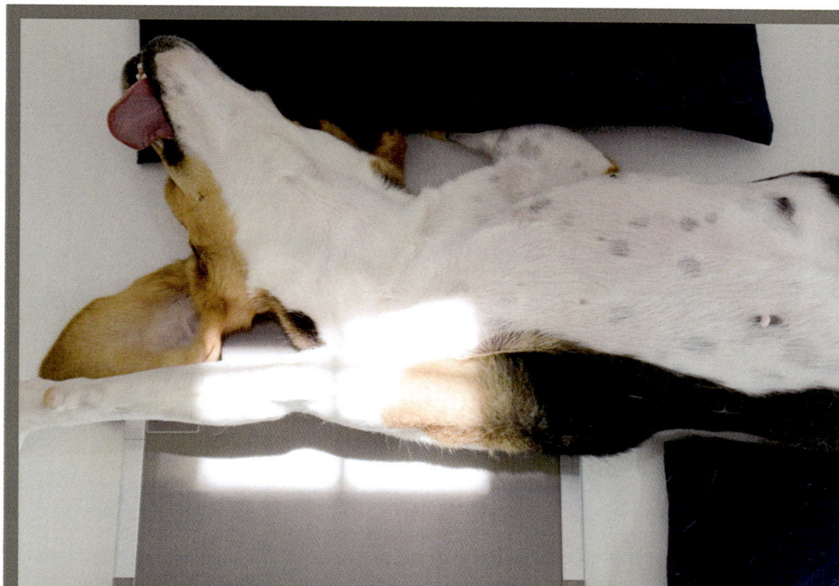

Fig. 17. In the caudocranial projection of the elbow, the X-ray beam should be centred on the distal end of the humerus.

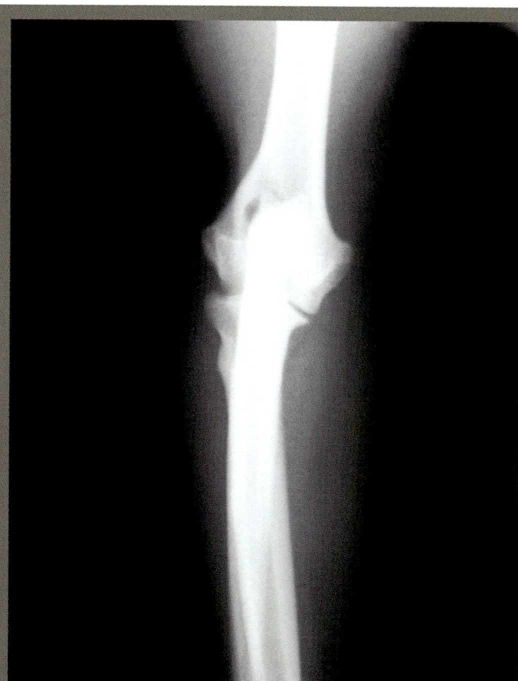

Fig. 18. Corresponding radiograph of CdCr projection of the elbow. ▶

In some situations, it may be more appropriate to use a **craniocaudal projection (CrCd)**. Examples are: assessment of **supra or intercondylar joint fractures of the humerus** or suspicion of incomplete intercondylar ossification (mainly in the American Cocker Spaniel).

For this projection:

- Place the sedated patient in dorsal recumbency.
- Pull the affected limb in caudal direction and fix it in traction.
- Turn the body slightly towards the affected side, so that the elbow does not superimpose on the thoracic cavity.
- Centre the primary beam on the intercondylar fossa of the humerus (Fig. 19).

In order to obtain a good radiographical image, the humerus should be aligned with the ulna and radius, which permits the best evaluation of the different areas of interest of the joint (Fig. 20).

If the condition is not very painful and the patient is quiet, it is possible to opt for a CrCd projection of the elbow with no need to sedate the patient.

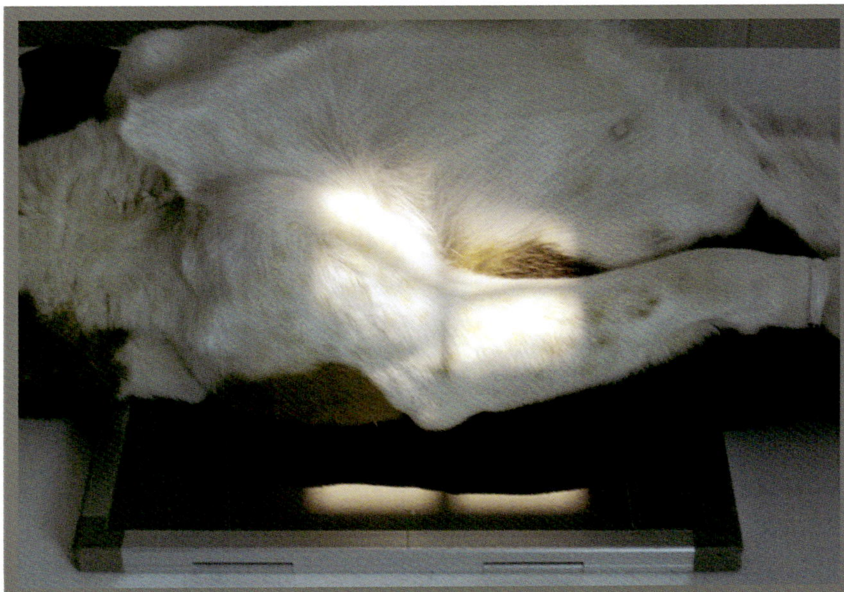

Fig. 19. Craniocaudal position of the elbow with no need to sedate the patient.

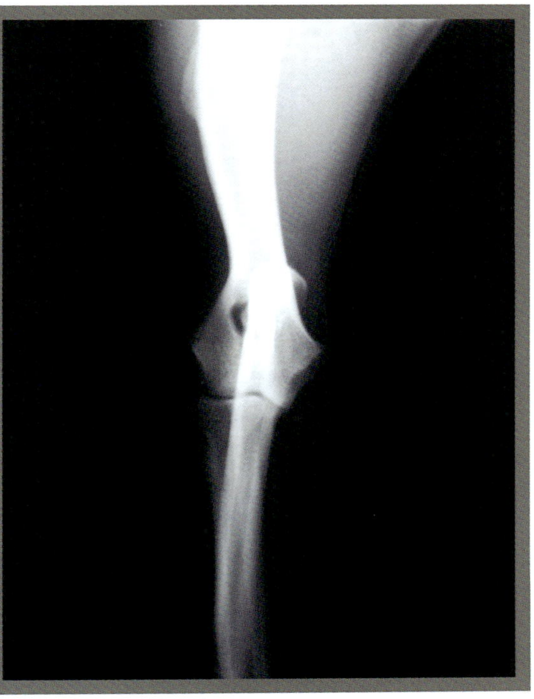

Fig. 20. Radiograph of the elbow in correct CrCd projection. ▶

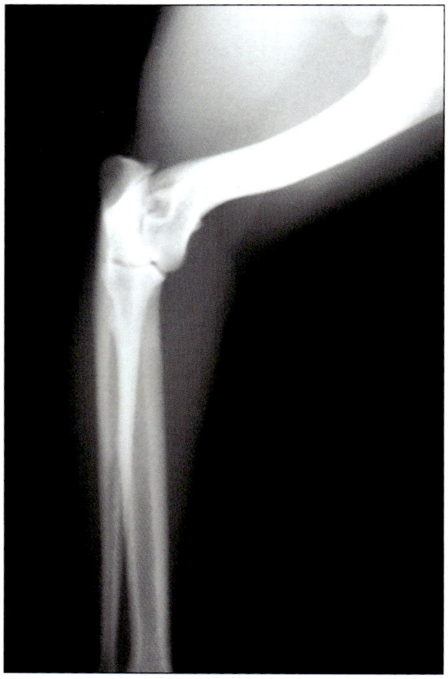

Fig. 21. Radiograph of the elbow in an incorrect CrCd projection.

If these steps are not followed, in particular the one concerning the correct alignment of the humerus and elbow, the image obtained will generally lack diagnostic quality (Fig. 21).

Apart from the projections that have been described, sometimes oblique projections are used, in particular the **caudomedial-craniolateral**, which, if correctly performed, allows visualization of the **fragmented medial coronoid process of the ulna** in cases of elbow dysplasia. However, in the authors' experience, what is usually diagnosed as fragmentation of the medial coronoid process is often no more than the formation of osteophytes around this area; still, this may indicate pathological changes.

Radius and ulna

To examine the lower limb, mediolateral and craniocaudal projections are used. As always, depending on the type of lesion and its painfulness, anything from a light sedation to general anaesthesia may be required.

For the **mediolateral (ML)** projection (Figs. 22 and 23):

- Place the patient in lateral recumbency with the affected side on the table.
- Pull the affected limb cranially and tie it down with the elbow in half-flexion.
- Include the proximal and the distal joint, that is, elbow and carpus, in the collimated image.
- Place a foam wedge under the foot to avoid rotation of the limb.
- Pull the other limb caudally and tie it back.
- Centre the primary beam on the central part of the diaphyses of the two bones.

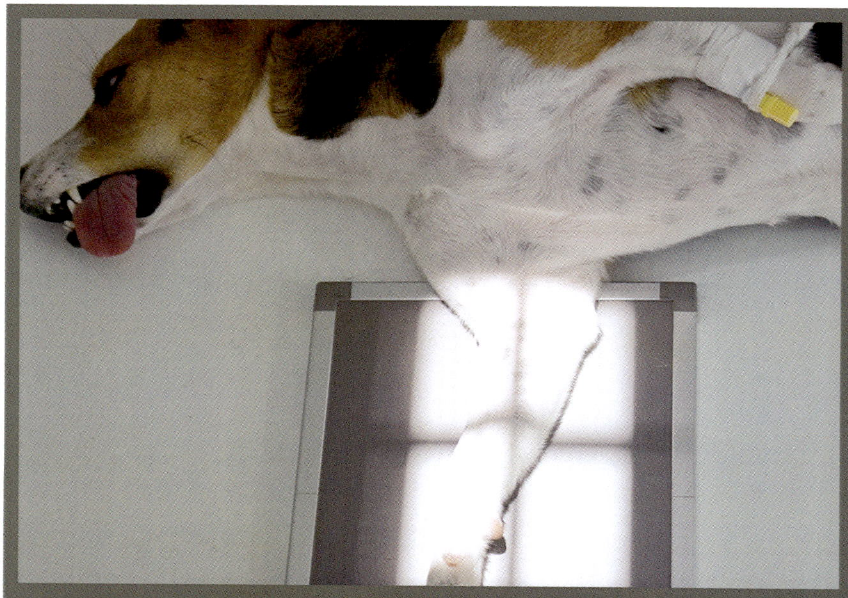

Fig. 22. Correct position for mediolateral projection of the ulna and radius.

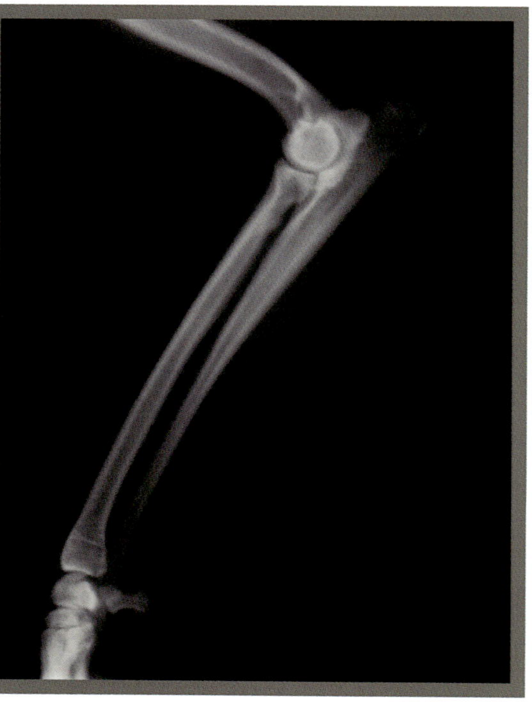

Fig. 23. Radiological image of the ML projection of the ulna and radius. ▶

This projection is very useful to assess the medullary cavity of the radius and ulna when suspecting **panosteitis**. It is also very effective for the diagnosis of traumatic **premature closure of the distal growth plates of the ulna and/or radius** and to assess the consequent deformations, if any.

The **craniocaudal (CrCd)** projection, perpendicular to the previous one, is the projection that is most commonly used. For this projection (Fig. 24):

- Place the patient in sternal recumbency.
- Place the head in extension on a foam aid to help maintain the position of the body.
- Pull the affected limb cranially and flex the healthy limb and raise it up to the level of the head.
- Use a foam wedge under the elbow to avoid slip or rotation.
- Rotate the body of the patient slightly in lateral direction to obtain good alignment of the whole area to be radiographed.
- Direct the primary beam towards the diaphyses of the radius and ulna.

This projection is very useful to diagnose **deviations of the limb due to premature closure of one or both distal growth plates**. It is also used to diagnose growth disturbances in pups of giant breeds, etc.

The CrCd projection of the radius and ulna is generally easy to perform and very useful to examine distal deviations in large or giant breeds.

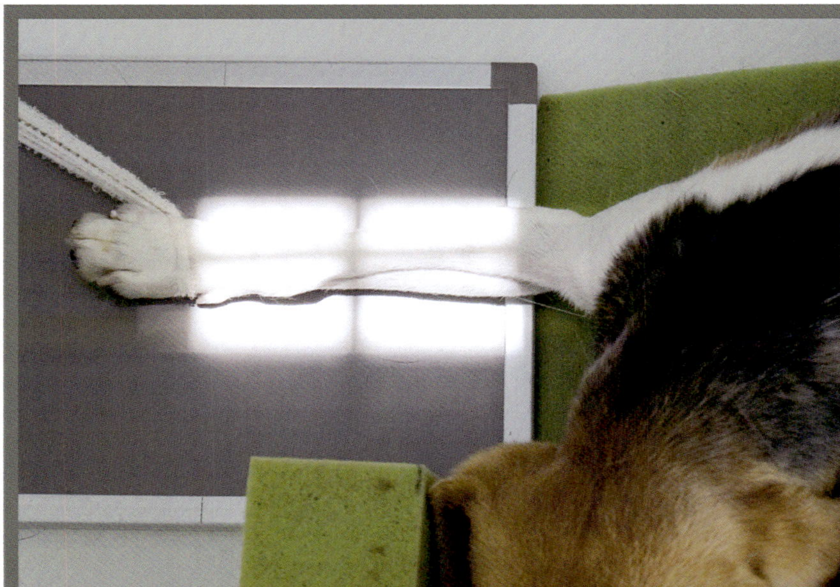

Fig. 24. Position of the limb for craniocaudal projection of the ulna and radius.

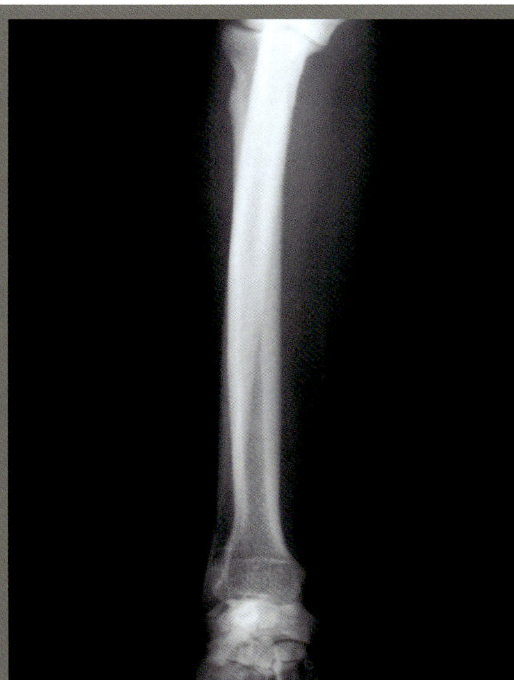

Fig. 25. Radiograph of the ulna and radius in CrCd projection. ▶

Carpus

Apart from the usual mediolateral (ML) and dorsopalmar (DP) projections, the so-called stress or forced projections are used for radiological examination of the carpus, to enable a correct assessment of the integrity of the many ligaments (collateral, dorsal, palmar, etc.) in this area.

For a **mediolateral (ML)** projection (Fig. 26):

- Place the patient in lateral recumbency with the affected side on the table.
- Pull the affected limb cranially and use a bandage or shoelace to fix it in this position.
- Pull the other limb out of the way in a caudal direction and tie it back.
- Place a radiolucent foam wedge under the foot to prevent the natural rotation of the area.
- Centre the primary beam on the base of the accessory carpal bone.

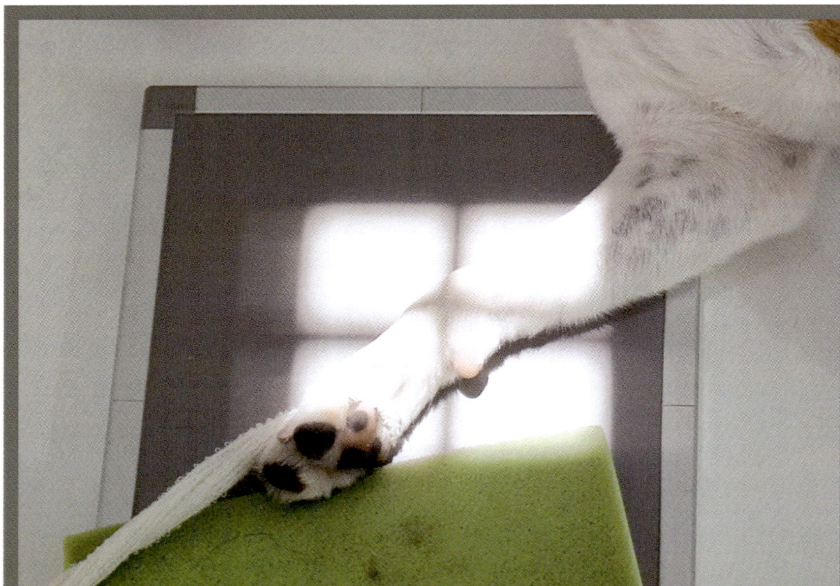

Fig. 26. Position of the limb to obtain a good radiograph of the carpus.

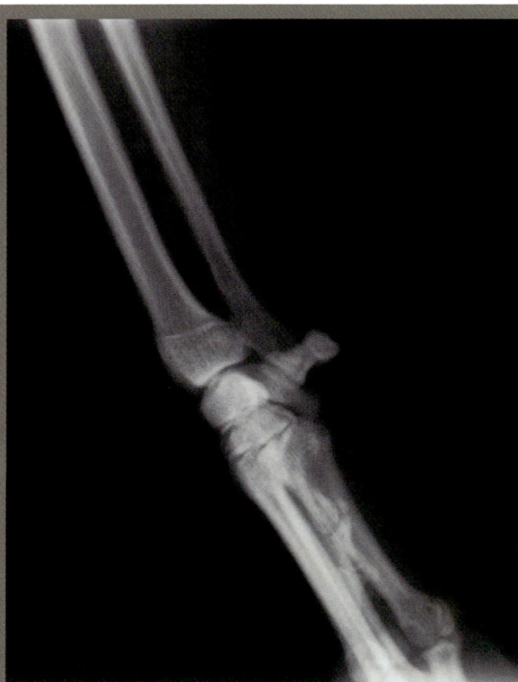

Fig. 27. ML radiograph of a well-positioned carpus. ▶

In this case, the position should be neutral, without applying force in any direction (Fig. 27). It allows the visualization of possible **fractures, dislocations or subluxations, periosteal reactions at the insertion area of the ligaments or inflammation of periarticular soft tissues**, which means that the radiograph should not be overexposed.

For **dorsopalmar (DP)** projection:

- Place the patient in sternal recumbency, with the head raised and supported by a square piece of foam to keep it in position.
- The affected limb is pulled cranially and fixed with a tie or bandage. Place a foam wedge under the elbow to ensure that it does not rotate and that the foot and carpus are parallel to the cassette and perpendicular to the beam.
- Place the other limb with the elbow in half flexion and raise it up to the level of the head to maintain the position of the body.
- Centre the primary beam on the accessory carpal bone.

It should be emphasised that for a truly diagnostic radiograph, the position should be perfect, because rotation of the carpus may lead to an erroneous diagnosis of fracture or subluxation that does not really exist. To obtain this position, it should be remembered that the carpus and the elbow should not be aligned, because that would cause rotation of the carpus.

Interpretation of the carpus is difficult due to the many joint lines, which is why the projection must be correct.

When suspecting rupture of ligaments, joint subluxation etc., stress or forced projections should be performed, for which the technique is the same as for the two previous projections, except that the joint is forced in extension with the aid of ties or bandages for the ML (Fig. 28) or DP (Fig. 29) projections.

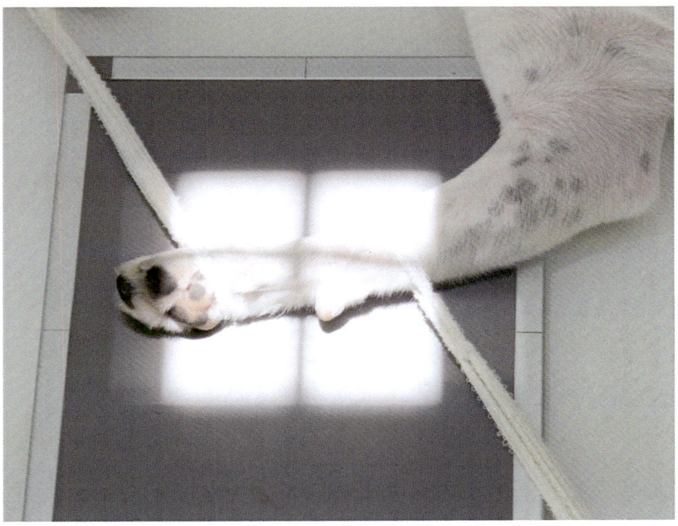

Fig. 28. Correct position for the mediolateral stress projection of the carpus.

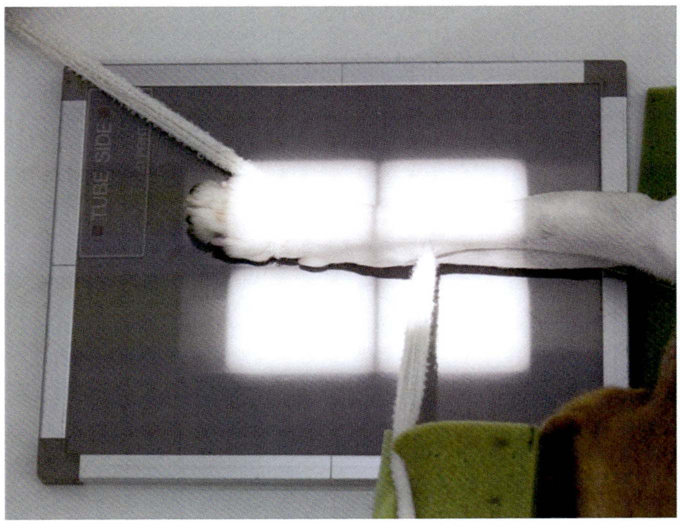

Fig. 29. Correct position for the dorsopalmar stress projection of the carpus.

The images obtained with the stress projections are compared with the normal images, which makes it possible to observe differences in the size of joint spaces, displacement of bone, etc.

In spite of all the projections mentioned above, it should be remembered that the carpus is an area of difficult radiological interpretation because of the presence of many joint lines that can confound the diagnosis.

Metacarpus and phalanges

In general, radiological examination of the metacarpus and phalanges is carried out using the same projections and positions as for the carpus. Differences or variations are:

- In mediolateral projection, the beam is centred on the metacarpo-phalangeal joint.
- Sometimes it is useful to use a slightly oblique projection to avoid superimposition of the bones (Figs. 30 and 31).

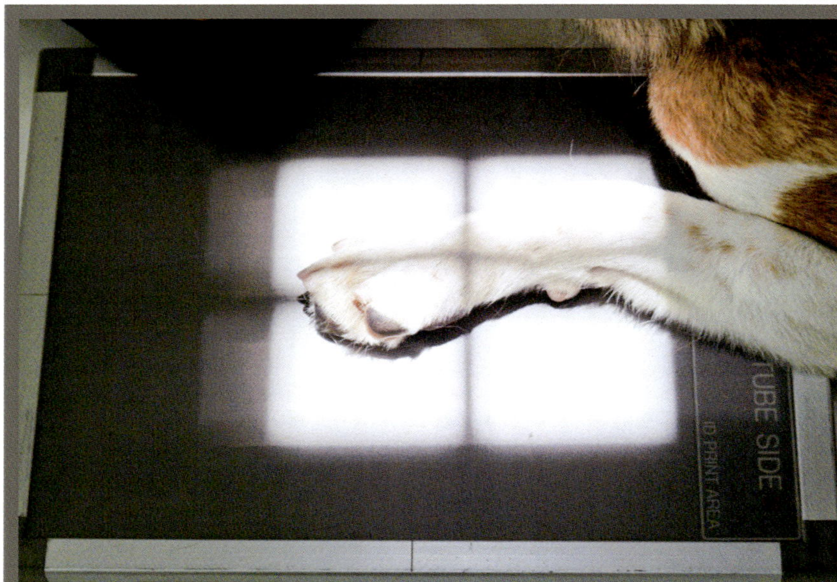

Fig. 30. Correct position for an oblique projection to radiograph the metacarpo-phalangeal area.

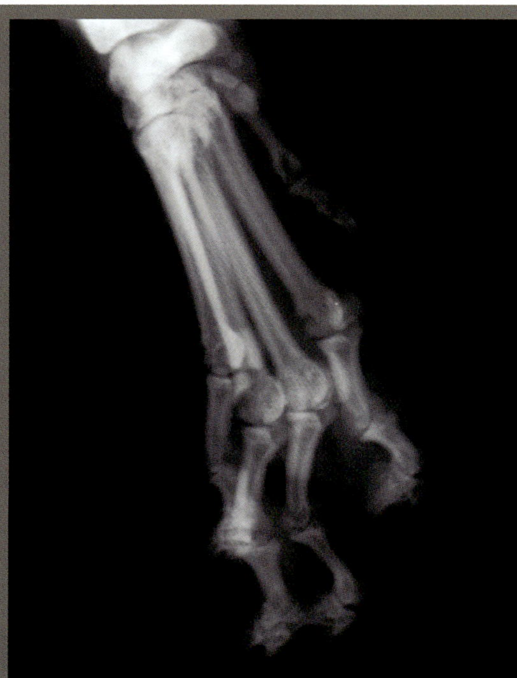

Fig. 31. Radiograph of the oblique projection in figure 30. ▶

For dorsopalmar projection it is useful to separate the toes with cotton wool pads or small foam wedges, so as to bring them into a symmetrical position.

A little dorsal pressure should be applied (Fig. 32) to bring the interphalangeal joints and the phalanges into the same position, so that they can be compared and checked for possible differences on the radiograph (Fig. 33).

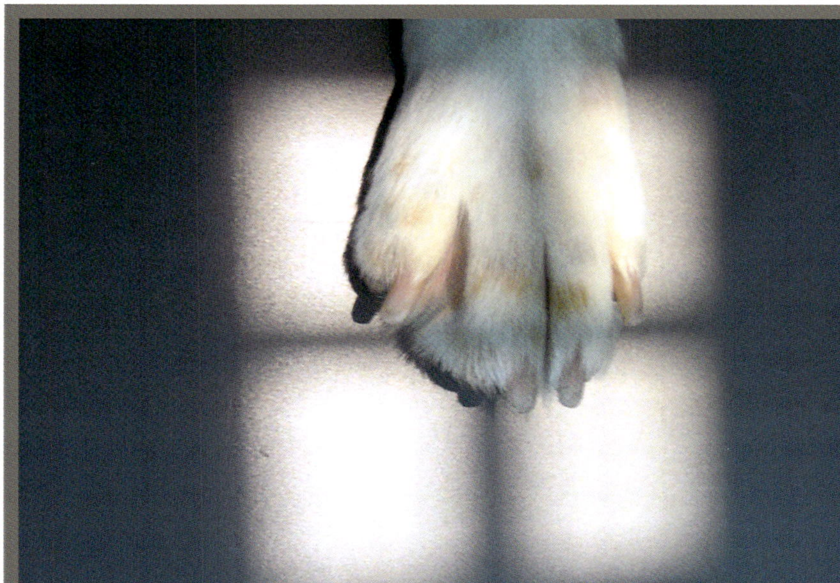

Fig. 32. Position applying dorsal pressure on the metacarpus and phalanges.

Fig. 33. Corresponding radiograph of the projection in figure 32. ▶

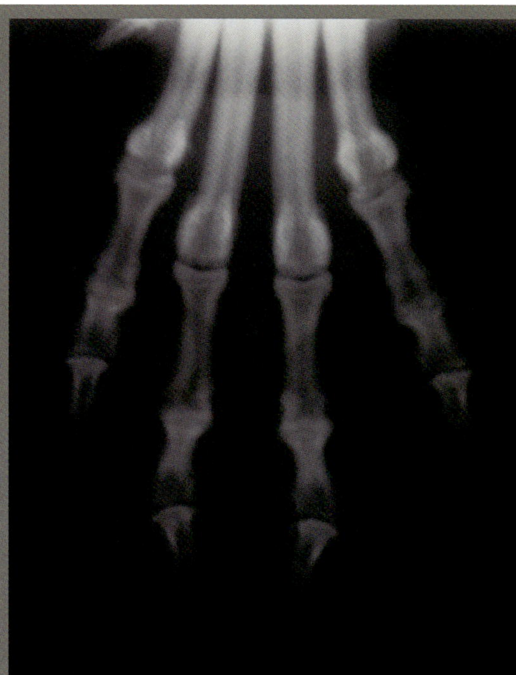

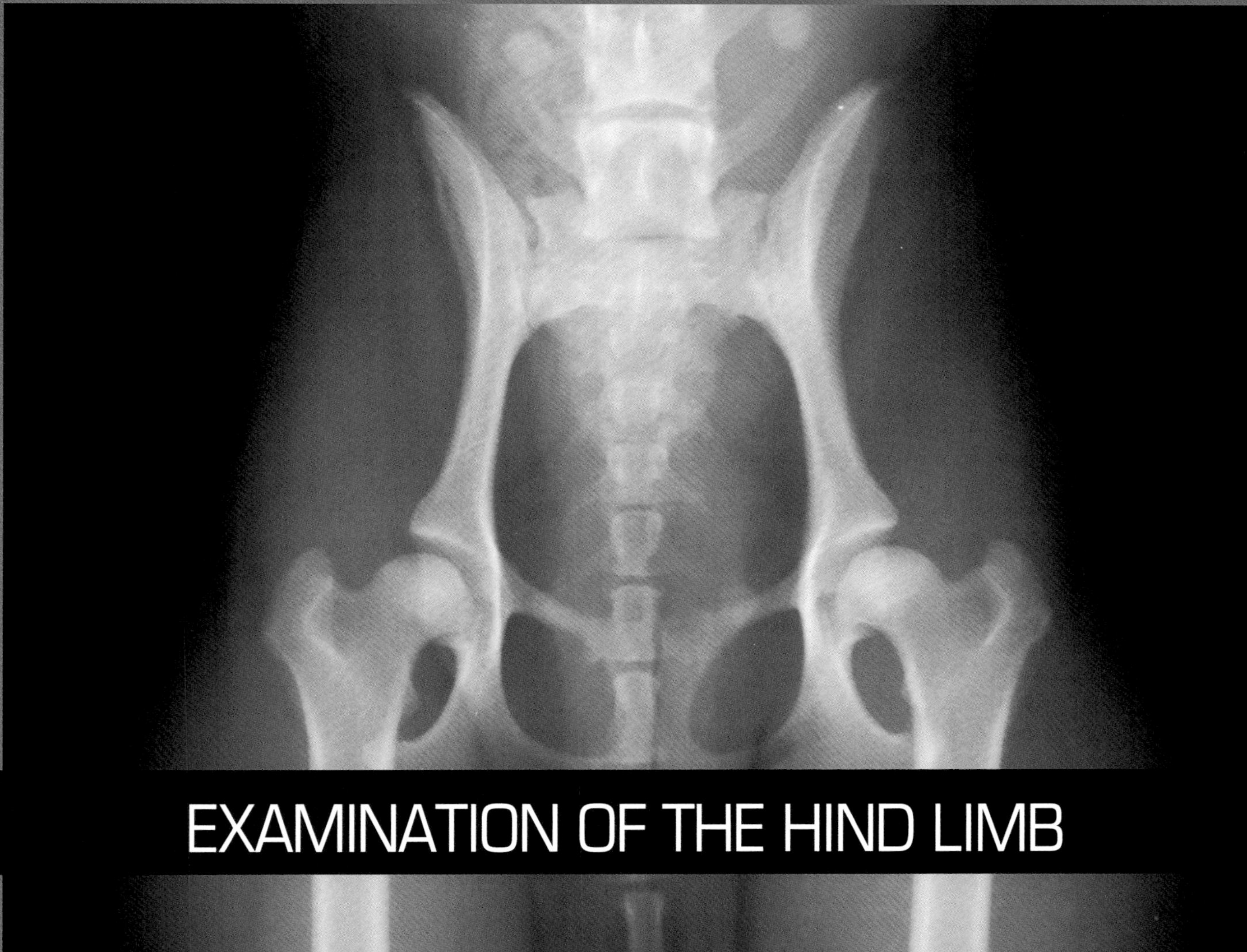

EXAMINATION OF THE HIND LIMB

General considerations

For radiological examination of the different areas of the hind limb, sedation of the patient is usually sufficient, except perhaps in case of severe pelvic trauma with fractures that may affect several bones and are usually very painful, so that deep sedation or general anaesthesia is often required. In these patients, the pre-anaesthetic assessment has to be very thorough, because there may be concurrent severe abdominal injury.

If general anaesthesia is required, extreme care should be taken because of the risk of concurrent severe abdominal injury.

In general, when examining the **pelvis**, including the sacrum and the caudal part of the spinal column, or the **femur** in heavily muscled dogs, an anti-scatter grid should be used, except in very small dogs, when the cassette can be placed directly on the table. For examination of the stifle or more distal structures, it is not necessary.

It should be highlighted in this chapter that the highest percentage of radiographic trauma investigations is carried out on the caudal third of the body, which tends to be the most commonly affected area in cases of trauma such as road traffic accidents.

Exposure factors

For examination of the pelvis and the coxo-femoral joint, **a relatively high mAs** should be used; it should always be higher in Lat projection than in VD, because this area is thicker in Lat projection. For the rest of the limb, 3 mAs is usually sufficient. The setting for the kV depends on the thickness of the area and varies from **45 to 75 kV**.

Positions and projections

To examine the different parts of the hind limb, at least two perpendicular projections should be obtained. The standard projections for the pelvis are the ventrodorsal (VD) and the lateral (Lat) projection. The mediolateral (ML) and the anterioposterior (AP) projections are most commonly used in the rest of the limb. The latter is called craniocaudal (CrCd) or caudocranial (CdCr) when referring to structures above the tarsus, and dorsoplantar (DPl) or plantarodorsal (PlD) when the tarsus itself or the structures distal to this joint are concerned. Apart from the projections mentioned above, several special projections will be described in the course of this chapter, in particular for the coxo-femoral joint, as this joint plays an important role in trauma cases and growth disturbances.

Next, each area with its peculiarities will be discussed, starting at the proximal end of the limb and ending with the phalanges.

Pelvis

Nowadays, radiological investigation of the pelvis represents a high proportion of the radiographs of the musculoskeletal system in veterinary practice, especially if the practice specialises traumatology and orthopaedics.

The projections that can be used are: standard ventrodorsal or ventrodorsal in extension (VD ext), ventrodorsal in frog position or in flexion (VD flex), lateral (Lat), tangential to assess the dorsal acetabular rim (DAR) and a projection called Penn Hip or forced distraction, which is not commonly used in Europe, because it requires a special distraction device designed by the University of Pennsylvania.

The most common projections to asses the pelvis are VD ext, VD flex, Lat and tangential or DAR.

For the **ventrodorsal projection in extension (VD ext),** these steps should be followed (Figs. 1 and 2):

- Place the patient in dorsal recumbency and maintain the position with a radiolucent wedge under its back.
- Secure the front of the animal by pulling both elbows symmetrically in a cranial direction, either manually or using sandbags.
- Apply firm traction to the hind limbs in a caudal direction, either manually or by means of bandages to which sandbags are tied as a counterweight.

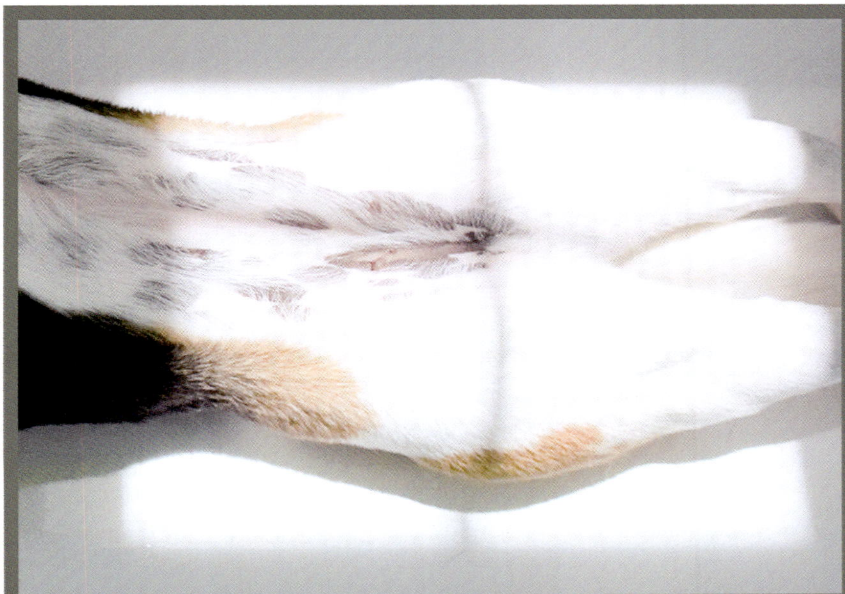

Fig. 1. Ventrodorsal position in extension to visualize the pelvis.

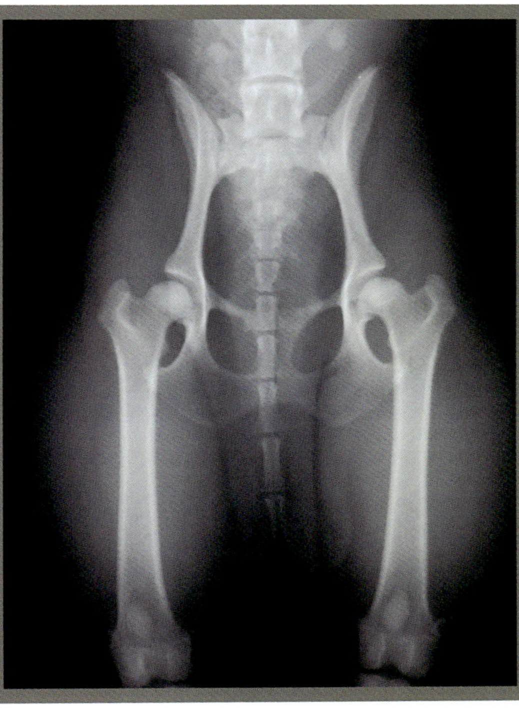

Fig. 2. Well-positioned radiograph obtained with the VD ext projection. ▶

- Keep the femurs parallel to each other and to the X-ray table, by applying traction to the hocks. If this is not done manually, it is advisable to tie a bandage around the stifles to rotate them towards the centre.
- Rotate both limbs inwards, in such a way that on the radiograph, the patellae are superimposed exactly on the trochlear groove, indicating an optimal position of the femur.
- Centre the primary beam on the imaginary line that joins the two greater trochanters of the femur.

When evaluating the radiograph obtained with this projection, it should be remembered that the superimposition of faeces and gas in the colon and rectum upon the bone structures may confound interpretation and lead to an erroneous diagnosis of pathological changes.

In male patients, the presence of the penile bone and the shadow of the prepuce, which is very radiopaque (Fig. 3), should also be kept in mind; they should not be mistaken for osteoclastic neoplasia.

Fig. 3. Radiograph of a male in which the penile bone (A) and the prepuce (B) can be observed.

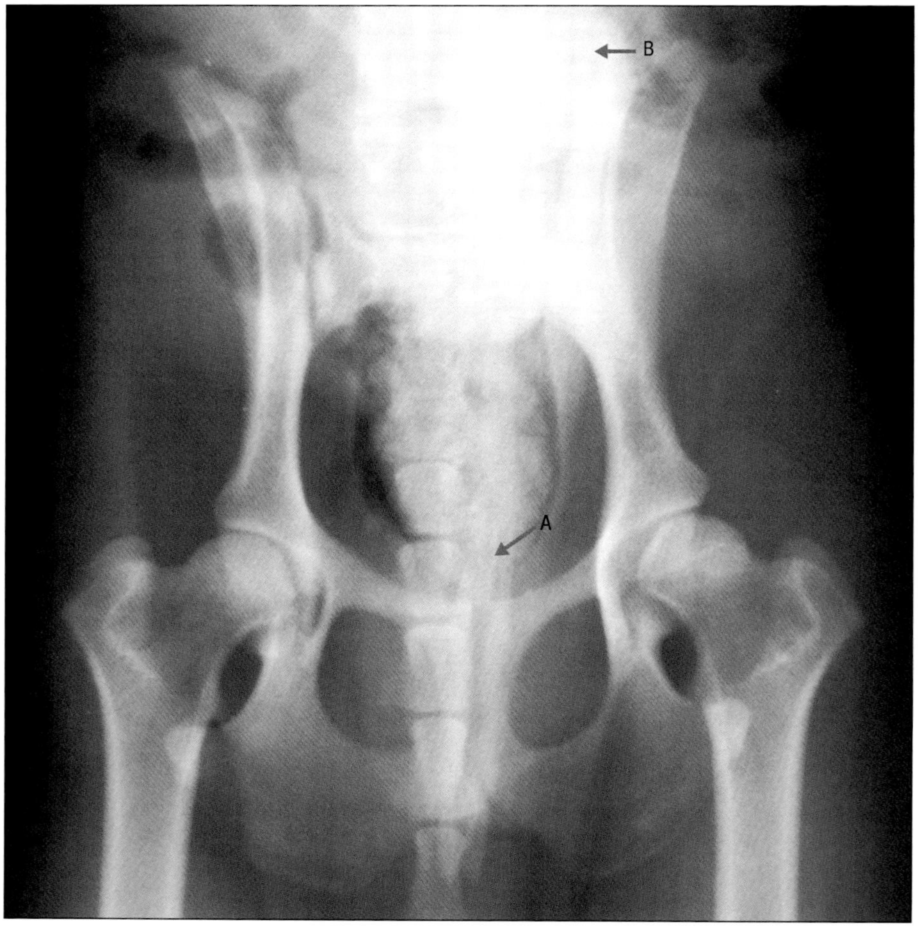

The VD in extension is usually the most suitable projection for assessing the degree of hip dysplasia and the consequent changes to the joint over time, in particular arthrosis.

For a **ventrodorsal projection in flexion (VD flex)** (Figs. 4 and 5):

- Place the patient in dorsal recumbency and maintain the position with a radiolucent wedge.
- Place sandbags on the axillae to maintain the position or apply manual traction to the elbows or axillae in a cranial direction.
- Flex both hips, stifles and hocks and maintain this position by either pushing the patient down on the X-ray table manually or by placing sandbags on the hocks, ensuring that both sides are symmetrical with regard to the centre of the beam.
- Centre the beam on the midpoint of the imaginary line between the two greater trochanters of the femurs.

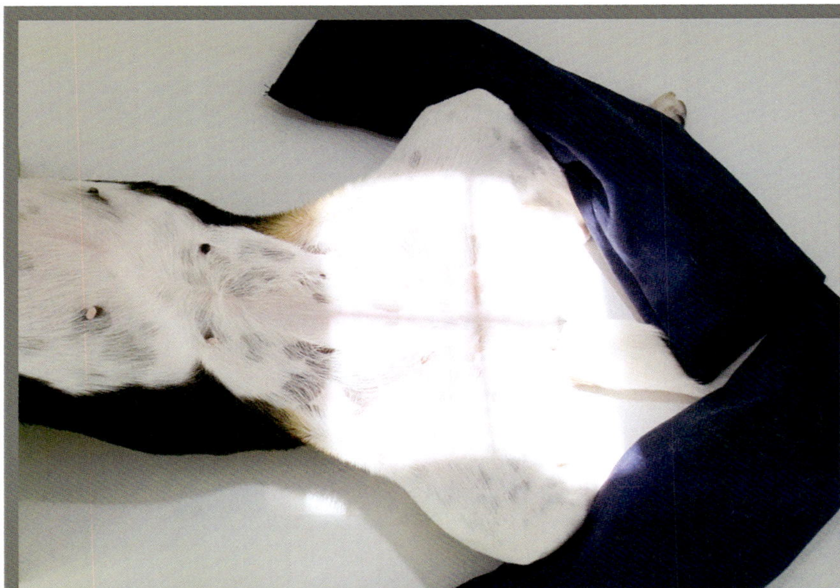

Fig. 4. Patient in dorsal recumbency with the hind limbs in flexion or "frog position".

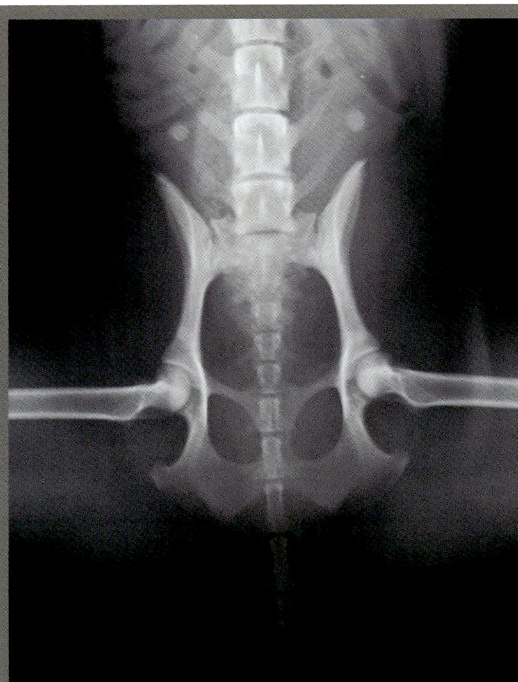

Fig. 5. Radiographic image of the pelvis in frog position. ▶

This projection is less painful than the VD in extension, which usually makes it easier to carry out in case of acetabular fracture or coxo-femoral dislocation, or when general anaesthesia is contraindicated. It is also very useful to assess joint congruity, even though the image obtained does not coincide with the physiological position of a standing animal.

As in the previous projection, it is helpful to evaluate the shape of the two **obturator foramina**, which should be as symmetrical as possible, to confirm that there is no rotation of the image with respect to the beam, because this could confound the diagnosis in case of suspected **hip dysplasia**.

For **lateral (Lat)** projection (Figs. 6 and 7):

- Place the animal in lateral recumbency, with the affected side on the table so that distortion is minimal, which is important when looking for small details on the radiograph.
- Apply traction to the hocks of both hind limbs in a caudal direction, either by hand or using bandages or ties.
- Place a foam aid or sandbag between the stifles to bring the two hind limbs parallel to each other and to the table.
- Apply traction to both forelimbs in a cranial direction, maintaining them in a parallel position.
- Avoid rotation of the sternum towards the table, in particular in patients with a deep thorax; a foam wedge placed underneath will help to maintain the correct position.

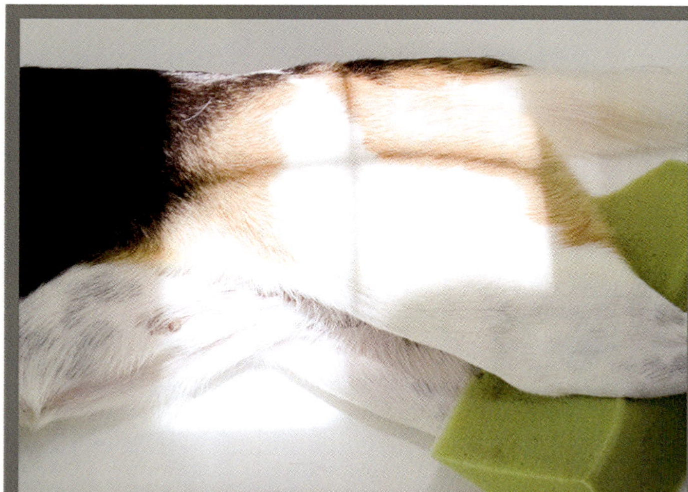

Fig. 6. Patient in lateral recumbency.

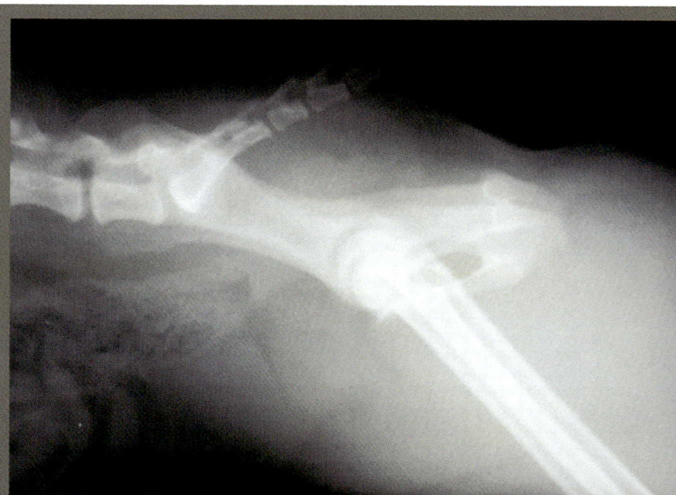

Fig. 7. Radiograph of the pelvis in Lat projection.

In cases of hip dysplasia, a so-called **tangential or DAR** (Dorsal Acetabular Rim) projection is used, which aims to assess the degree of acetabular coverage in a position that is as similar as possible to that of a standing animal, in preparation for a triple pelvic osteotomy or a total hip replacement. This is a special projection for which it is necessary to sedate or anaesthetise the animal, because it is uncomfortable and may cause a certain amount of distress to the patient.

For this projection:

- Place the patient in sternal recumbency and use a radiolucent wedge to avoid rotation.
- Keep the forelimbs close to the body, slightly flexed at the elbow.
- Place a foam positioning aid, if possible cylindrical, under the cervical column to keep the head and neck in a raised position.
- Pull both hind limbs cranially and keep them close to the body with a bandage or tie. Sometimes foam aids are placed under the hocks to improve the position.
- Centre the primary beam on the midpoint between the greater trochanters of the femurs; if the X-ray tube is mobile, it should be rotated by 15 degrees in a cranial direction to obtain an even better projection (Figs. 8, 9 and 10).

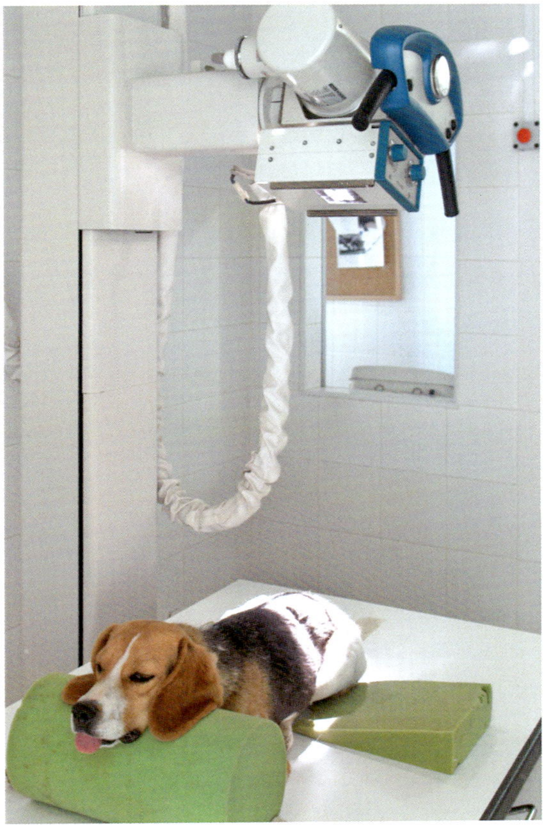

Fig. 8. Position for the tangential or DAR projection, frontal view.

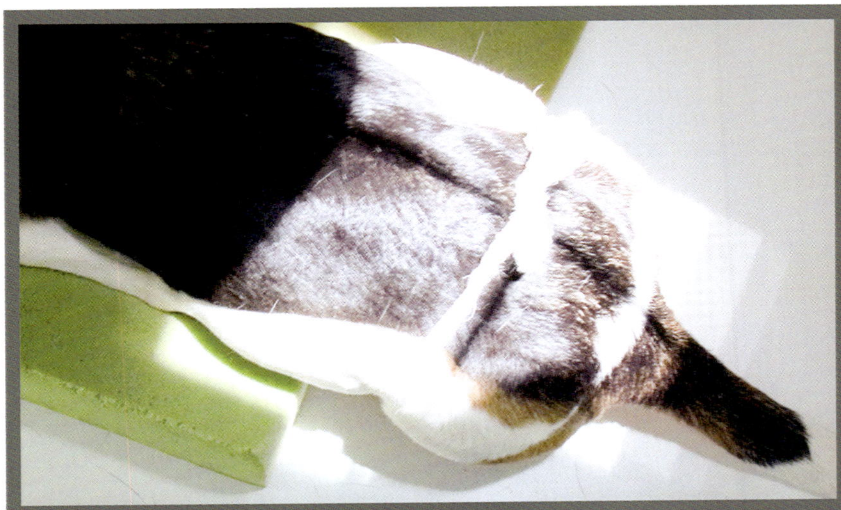

Fig. 9. Correct positioning for the tangential or DAR projection of the pelvis, seen from above.

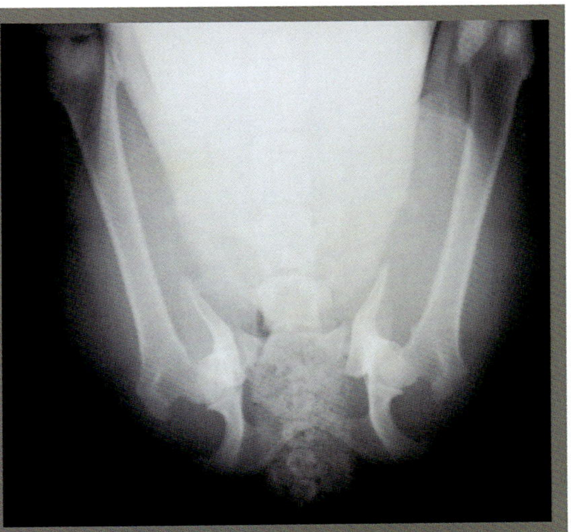

Fig. 10. Radiograph of the pelvis obtained with the tangential projection.

Femur

Radiological examination of the femur requires two perpendicular projections, such as the mediolateral (ML) and caudocranial (CdCr). It can also be examined in the VD ext projection of the pelvis that has been described, but in this case, the limb is further from the X-ray table and the film, which is why the CdCr projection gives a more representative image of the size and shape of the femur.

For a good radiograph of the femur in **mediolateral (ML) projection** (Figs. 11 and 12):

- Place the patient in lateral recumbency with the affected limb against the table.
- Pull the healthy limb back or lift it up, and keep it in position with a bandage or tie.
- Keep the affected limb in half-flexion, without forcing extension, as near as possible to the position in a standing animal.
- Avoid rotation of the limb by placing a foam wedge under the hock and foot.
- Centre the X-ray beam on the central part of the femoral diaphysis, including both the proximal part of the femur and the condyles in the radiograph.
- In most cases, an anti-scatter grid should be used to reduce scattered radiation.

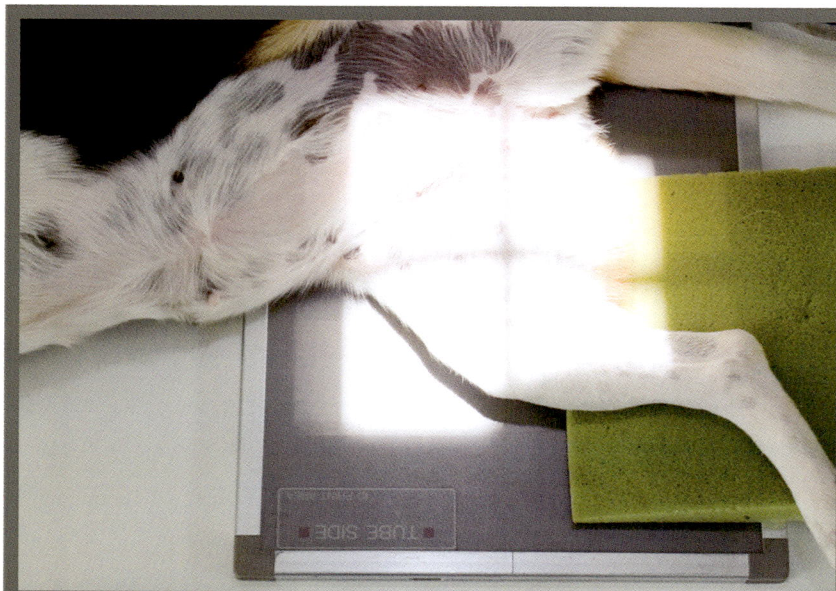

Fig. 11. Correct position for the mediolateral projection of the femur.

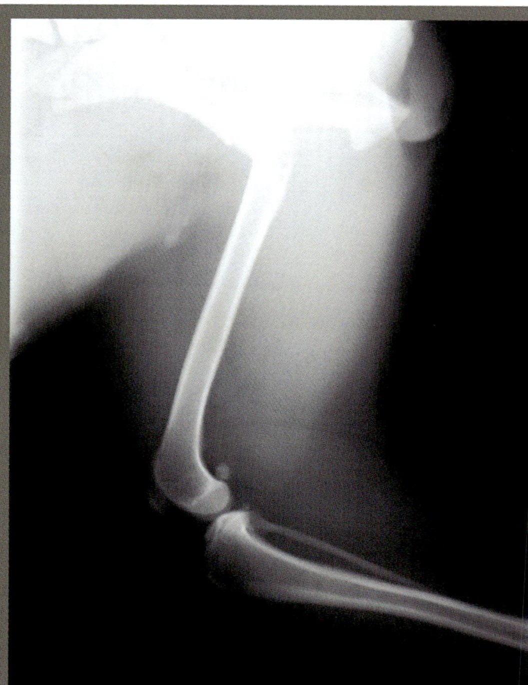

Fig. 12. The radiographic image obtained with the ML projection should be similar to this one. ▶

For a good image in **caudocranial (CdCr) projection** (Figs. 13 and 14):

- Place the patient in sternal recumbency and maintain the position with a wedge under the thorax or with sandbags in the flanks.
- Pull the affected limb caudally and rotate it slightly in a medial direction, so that the patella remains in the patellar groove. To maintain this position, a foam pad can be placed under the stifle, or else the tarsus and tibiofibular area can be weighted down with sandbags.
- Keep the other limb flexed, so that it does not interfere with the image, and slightly elevated on a rectangular foam pad, which also helps to maintain the position of the animal.
- Rotate the body slightly towards the affected side.
- Centre the beam on the central area of the femoral diaphysis.

For a good radiograph of the femur in CdCr projection, it is essential to prevent axial rotation; this is achieved by placing a foam pad under the stifle.

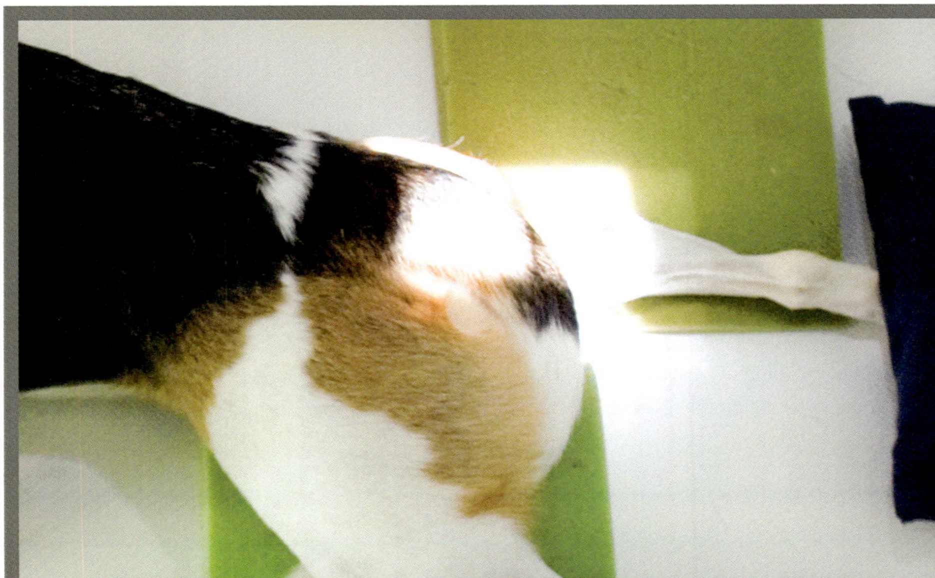

Fig. 13. Position for the caudocranial projection for examination of the femur.

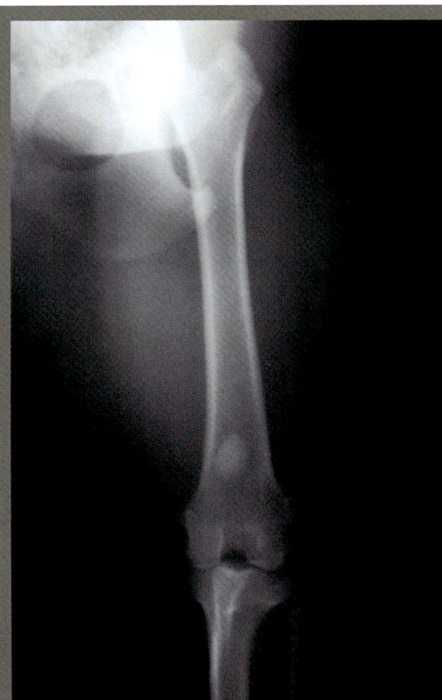

Fig. 14. Radiograph of the femur in CdCr projection. ▶

Stifle

The stifle joint is another area that is examined very frequently, because many patients in veterinary practice present with stifle problems. Therefore, good projections are indispensable to reach a correct diagnosis.

The mediolateral and caudocranial projections are most commonly used for examination of the stifle; occasionally, in patients with patellar luxation, the skyline or horizontal beam projection is used, which enables evaluation of the depth of the trochlear groove.

As discussed in the general considerations, for none of these projections it is necessary to use an anti-scatter grid, as the thickness is never more than 10 or 12 cm.

For a good **mediolateral (ML)** projection (Figs. 15 and 16):

- Place the patient in lateral recumbency with the affected limb against the table. The stifle and tarsus should be in half-flexion, as near as possible to the position of a standing animal.
- Pull the other limb cranially without using excessive force to avoid rotation and secure it in this position with a bandage.
- Place a foam wedge under the hock to keep the stifle perfectly parallel to the primary beam.
- Centre the X-ray beam on the distal area of the femoral condyles.

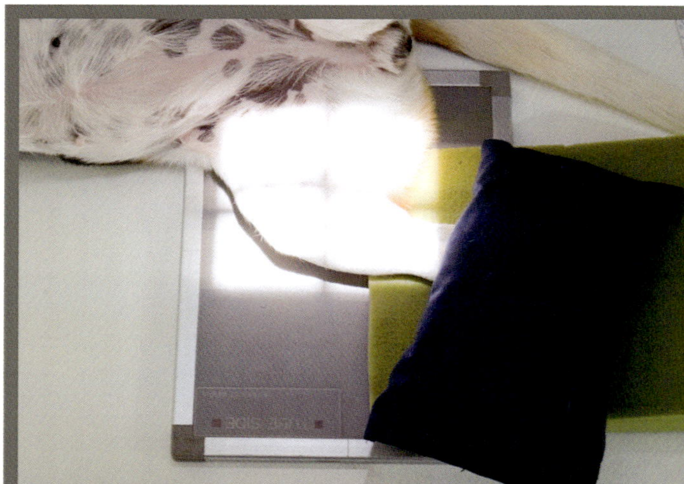

Fig. 15. Correct position for a mediolateral projection of the stifle, one of the most commonly used in orthopaedic radiography.

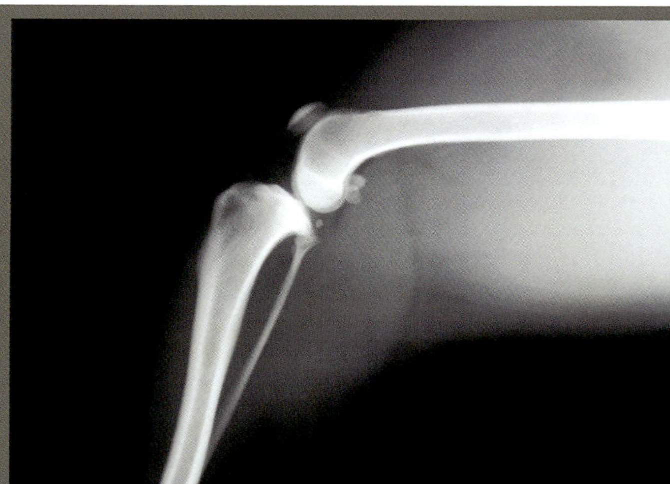

Fig. 16. To obtain a ML radiograph with diagnostic value, the femoral condyles should be perfectly superimposed.

In mediolateral projection of the stifle, superimposition of the femoral condyles is indispensable to evaluate if there is joint effusion and to plan certain surgical techniques.

When carrying out this projection, there is often a tendency to pull the healthy limb back in a caudal direction because that seems to be easier; however, in that position it is much more difficult to obtain perfect superimposition of the femoral condyles. And that is indispensable for adequate assessment of the presence or absence of joint effusion, as well as carrying out the necessary **measurements** when planning a tibial plateau levelling osteotomy for cruciate ligament rupture. In the latter case, the hock joint should also be included in the radiograph.

For **caudocranial (CdCr)** projection of the stifle (Figs. 17 and 18):

- Place the patient in sternal recumbency with the affected limb pulled perfectly straight in a caudal direction.
- Flex and raise the other limb by means of a rectangular foam pad.
- Place a foam wedge under the affected stifle in such a way that the patella is not in contact with the cassette, and centred in the trochlear groove.
- Rotate the body slightly towards the affected side.
- Centre the X-ray beam on the distal part of the patella.

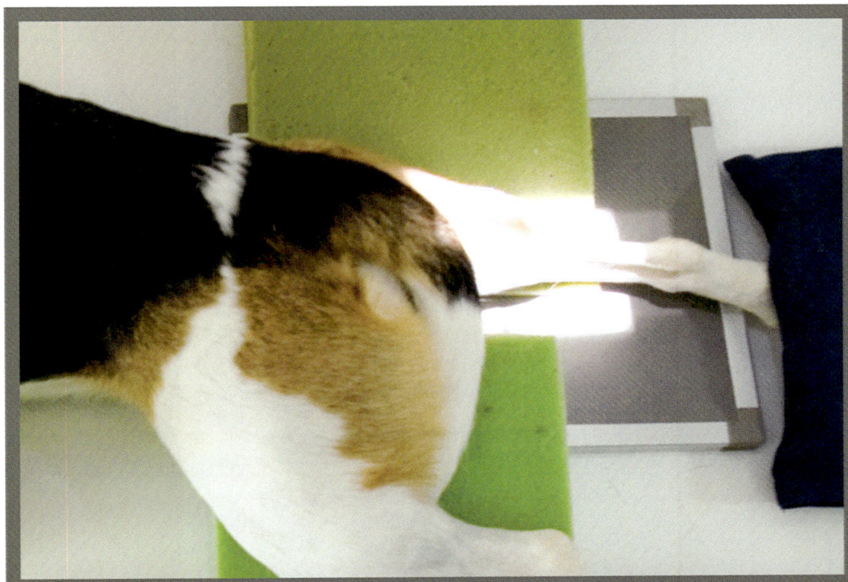

Fig. 17. Patient in the correct position for caudocranial projection of the stifle.

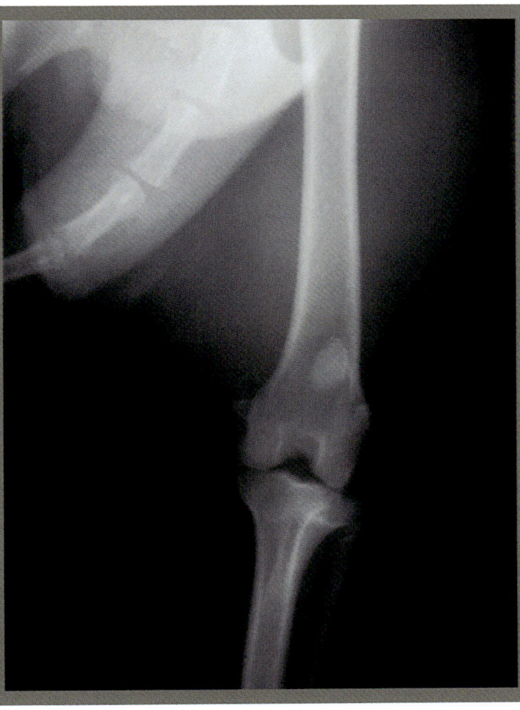

Fig. 18. The CdCr projection results in a better radiograph than the CrCd projection, because the stifle is resting on the cassette in a perfect position. ▶

When evaluating the depth of the trochlear groove for surgery in case of patellar luxation, a **skyline or horizontal beam projection** can be used, for which the X-ray tube needs to be mobile in several directions.

For this projection:

- Place the patient in dorsal recumbency and maintain the position with a foam wedge or sandbags against the flanks.
- Flex the stifle until the patella reaches its highest position. This has to be done manually by gripping the tarsus, so careful protective measures should be taken.
- Place the cassette in a vertical position, either leaning on the inguinal area of the patient or held up manually by an assistant.
- Move the X-ray tube in a caudal direction, rotate it 90° cranially and bring it down towards the table so that the beam hits the patella and patellar groove tangentially. The distance between the cassette and the X-ray tube should be about one metre.
- Centre the primary beam on the patella.

In this projection there is hardly any soft tissue, so the kilovoltage should be reduced considerably, because if not, the image will be overexposed (Figs. 19, 20 and 21).

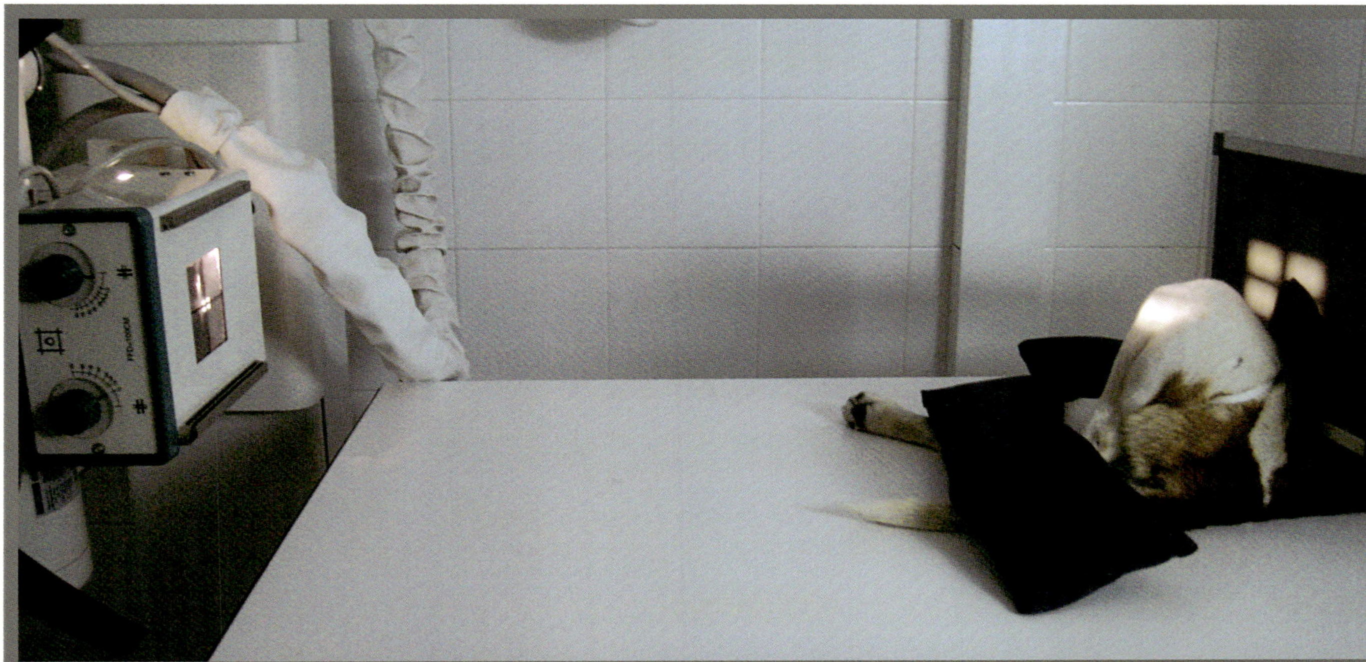

Fig. 19. Lateral view of the position for the tangential or skyline projection, to visualize the patella and the patellar groove.

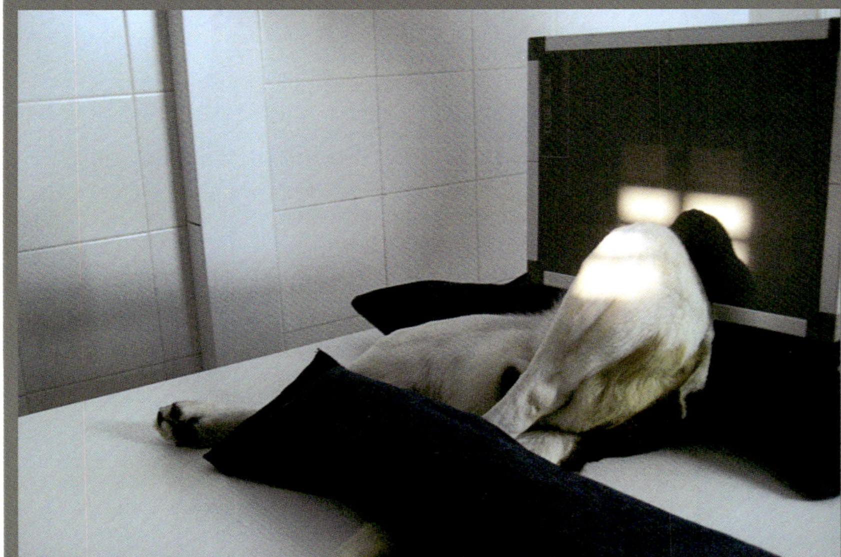

Fig. 20. Dorsal view of the position for the tangential or skyline projection, to visualize the patella and the patellar groove.

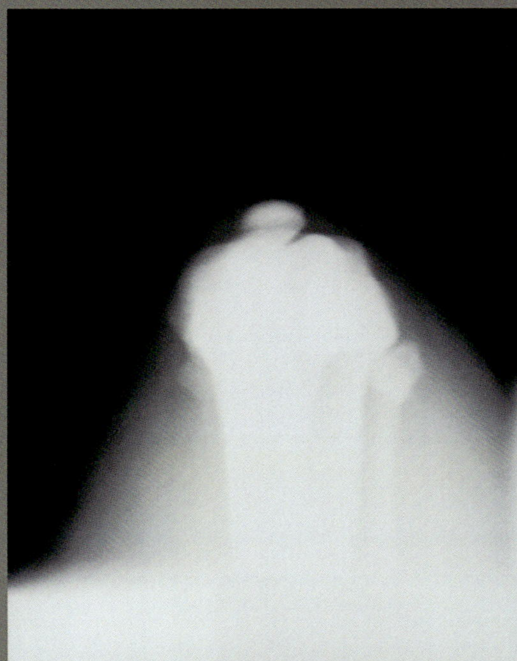

Fig. 21. Radiograph obtained with tangential projection of the patella. ▶

Tibia and fibula

To carry out a good examination of the tibia and fibula, two perpendicular projections, such as the mediolateral and caudocranial, usually suffice. As there is little muscle mass around this area, the quality and contrast of the images obtained is good; compared to other parts of the hind limb, a low setting for the kilovoltage should be used even in heavily muscled dogs.

For a good image in **mediolateral (ML)** projection:

- Place the patient in lateral recumbency, with the affected limb on the cassette.
- Pull the other limb cranially without excessive force to avoid rotation, and maintain it in position with a bandage.
- Place a foam wedge under the tarsus, so that the tibia and fibula remain perfectly parallel to the radiographic cassette.
- Centre the X-ray beam on the central part of the diaphyses of the two bones (Fig. 23).

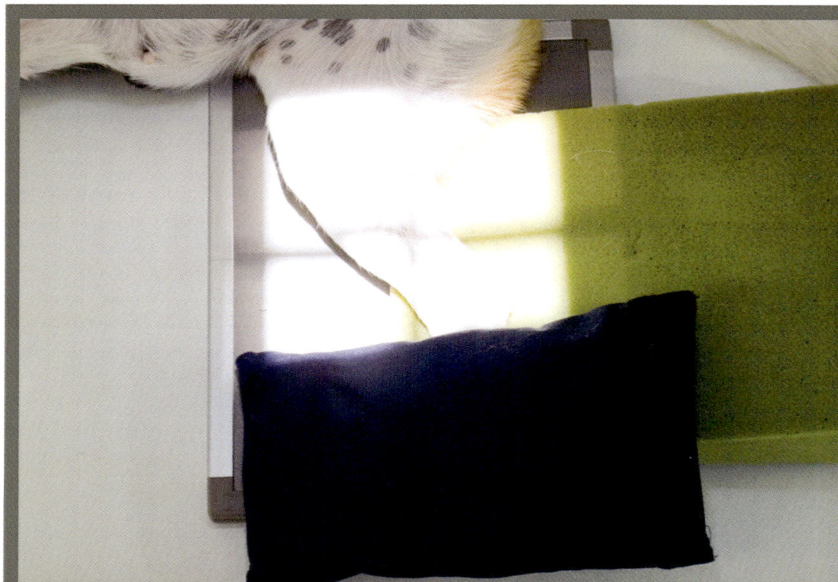

Fig. 22. Position for the mediolateral projection of the tibia and fibula, including the stifle and hock.

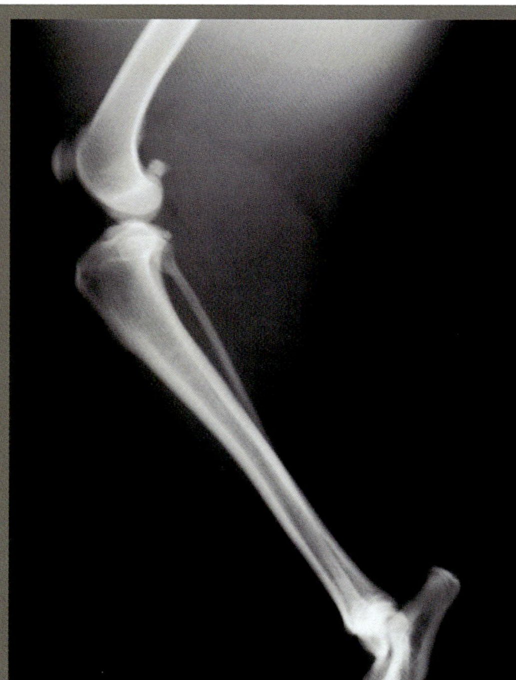

Fig. 23. Radiographic image of the tibia and fibula obtained with the ML projection. ▶

In the mediolateral projection of the tibia and fibula, the proximal and distal joints should be included; this makes it possible to carry out measurements for corrective interventions.

With this projection, it is often necessary to include both the proximal joint (stifle) and the distal joint (tarsus), as it is necessary to obtain a complete image of both bones (Fig. 22) to carry out measurements and calculate angles for subsequent interventions (for instance in case of angular deformities or tibial plateau levelling).

For a good image in **caudocranial (CdCr)** projection (Figs. 24 and 25):

- Place the patient in sternal recumbency, with the affected limb pulled perfectly straight in a caudal direction.
- Flex and raise the other limb with a rectangular piece of foam.
- Place a foam wedge under the stifle of the affected limb in such a way that the patella does not make contact with the cassette, which will avoid rotation of the limb.
- Rotate the body slightly towards the affected side.
- Centre the X-ray beam on the central part of the diaphyses of the tibia and fibula.

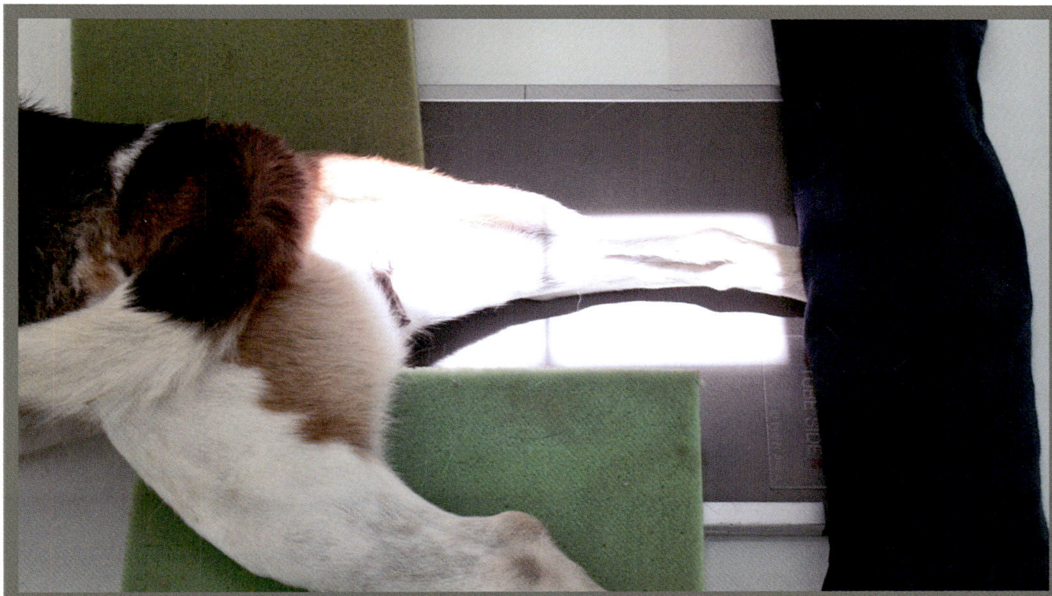

Fig. 24. Position for the caudocranial projection for examination of the tibia and fibula.

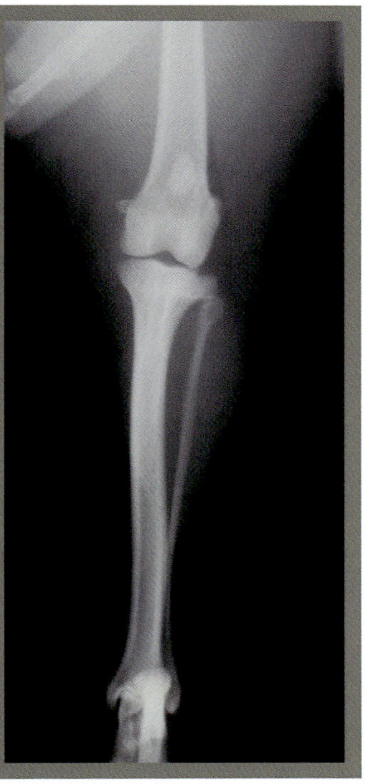

Fig. 25. Radiograph of the tibia and fibula in CdCr projection. ▶

Tarsus (hock)

Radiographic investigation of the tarsus can nearly always be carried out with the two perpendicular projections that have been discussed in this chapter, the mediolateral and the caudocranial (called plantarodorsal in this case), as well as the stressed or forced projections that have been discussed for examination of the carpus.

However, on some occasions, such as in growing dogs of large or giant breeds, a special projection is needed for correct visualization of the articular surface of the talus bone without any superimposition of other bony structures, to look for possible lesions of osteochondrosis or osteochondritis dissecans. This is the tangential projection of the tarsus, which will be described later on.

For a **mediolateral (ML)** projection of the tarsus (Figs. 26 and 27), the steps to be followed are the same as for the stifle or tibia, but in this case the X-ray beam should be centred distal to the tibio-tarsal joint.

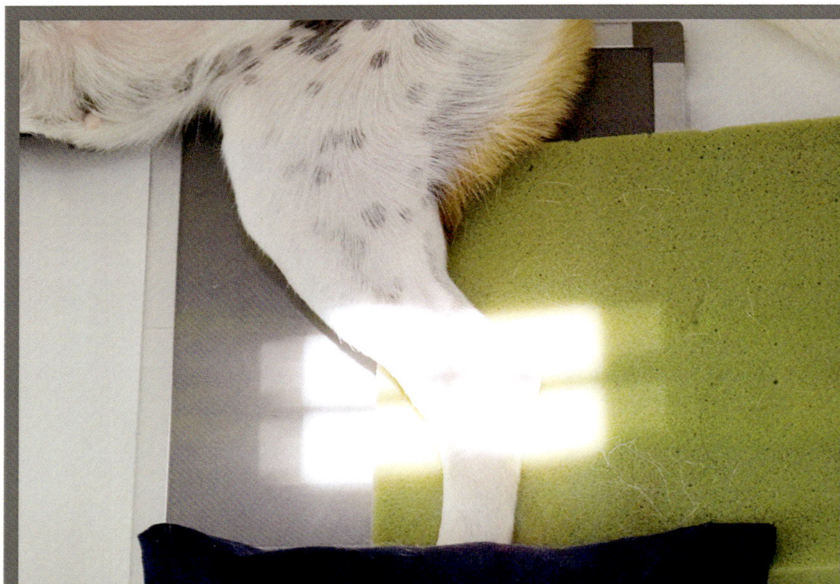

Fig. 26. Position for the mediolateral projection of the tarsus.

Fig. 27. Well-positioned radiograph for investigation of the tarsus, which is difficult. ▶

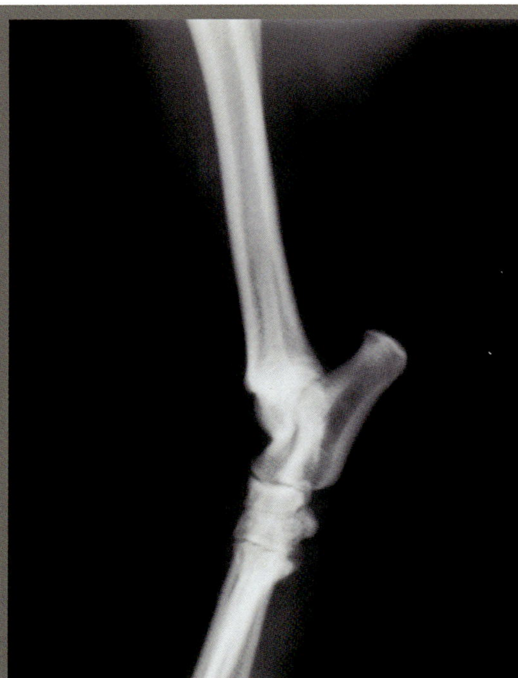

For the **plantarodorsal (PlD)** projection, the procedure is also the same as for the stifle or the tibia, but once more, the X-ray beam is centred distal to the tibio-tarsal joint (Figs. 28 and 29).

For stress or forced projections to assess the integrity of the main ligaments that stabilise the tarsus, bandages or ties can be used to apply traction in whatever direction, without having to expose any part of the radiographer or assistants to the primary radiation in the X-ray room.

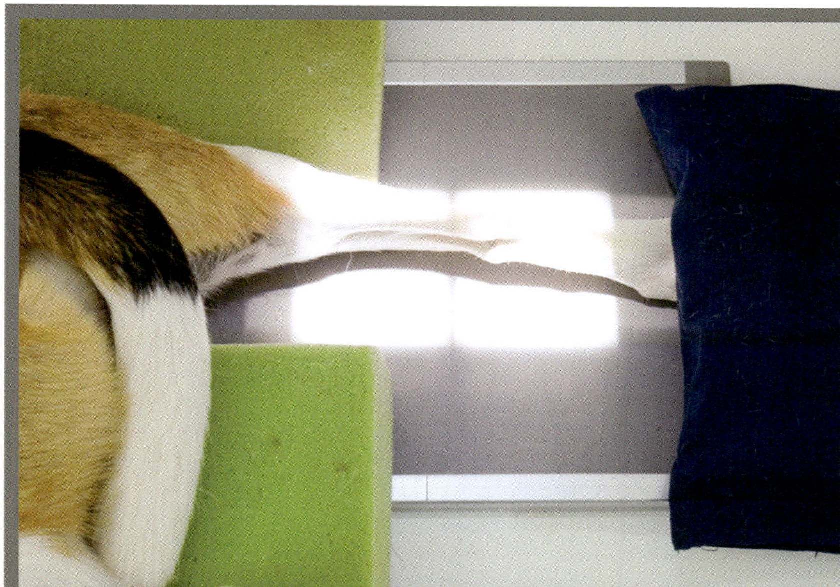

Fig. 28. Correct position for the plantarodorsal projection of the tarsus.

Fig. 27. Radiographic image of the projection in Fig. 28. ▶

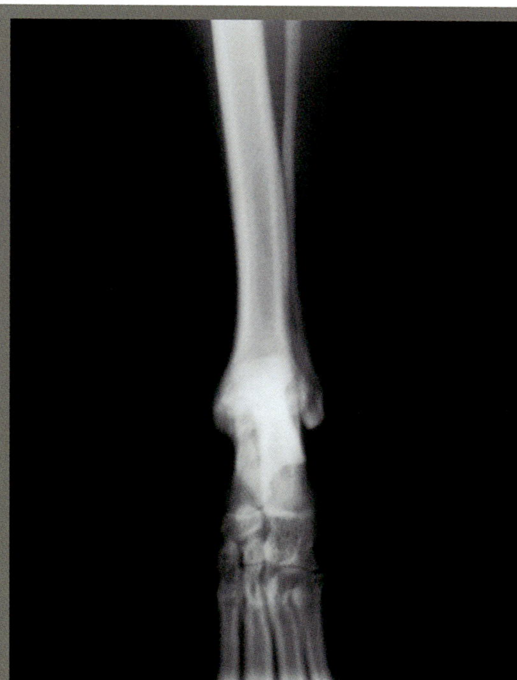

The tangential projection of the tarsus makes it possible to evaluate lesions caused by osteochondrosis or osteochondritis dissecans of the talus bone in patients of large or giant breeds.

As has been mentioned, sometimes patients of large or giant breeds present lameness due to tarsal problems. To confirm a suspected osteochondrosis or osteochondritis dissecans of the talus bone, the **skyline projection of the tarsus** (Figs. 30 and 31) should be used. For this projection:

- Place the patient in dorsal recumbency with a wedge under its back to maintain the position.
- Flex both the stifle and the tarsus of the affected limb in a 90° angle.
- Place a cassette on a rectangular piece of foam at the level of the tibia and tarsus and place the affected joint on it.
- If the X-ray tube is mobile, it is raised up until the distance between the radiographic cassette and tube is one metre.
- Move the tube in a cranial direction and rotate it slightly caudally, in such a way that the X-ray beam hits the articular surface of the talus bone tangentially, without superimposition of the calcaneal tuberosity.

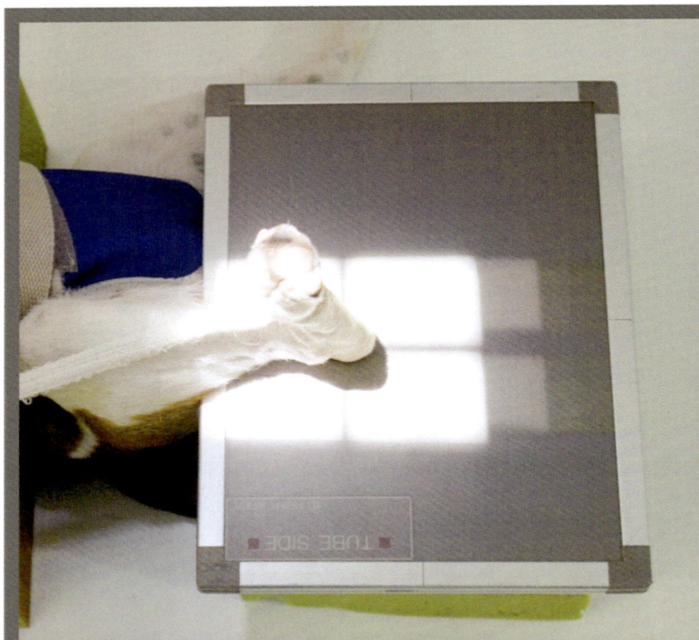

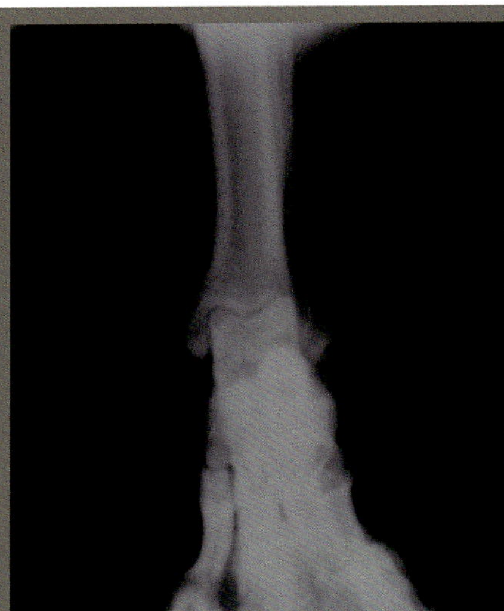

▲ Fig. 31. The radiograph allows evaluation of the complete articular surface of the talus bone.

Fig. 30. The tangential projection of the tarsus requires a special position of the patient, as shown in this picture.

With this projection, superposition of the calcaneal tuberosity on the lateral malleolus of the talus bone is avoided, which is the side that is usually affected by these pathological processes.

Metatarsus and phalanges

Generally, examination of the distal part of the hind limb requires only the two main projections (mediolateral and plantarodorsal) that have been used in the last few paragraphs.

Both can be carried out positioning the affected limb as for the ML and CdCr projections of the tarsus, but displacing the primary beam distally to coincide with the metatarsophalangeal joints (Figs. 32 and 33).

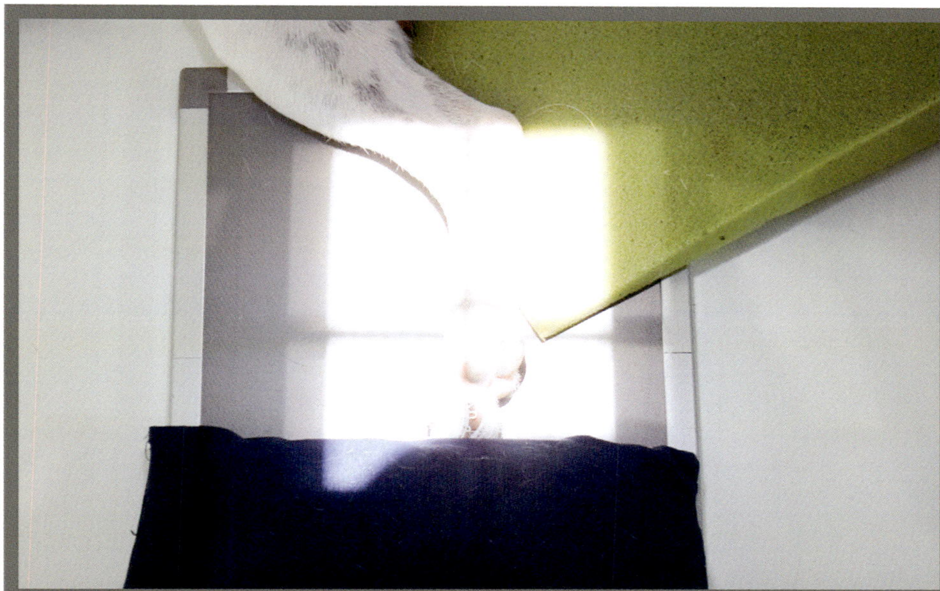

Fig. 32. Position for the mediolateral projection of the metatarsus and the phalanges.

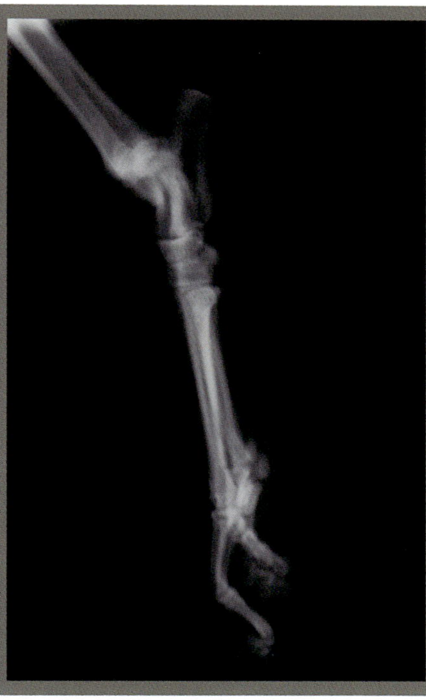

Fig. 33. Radiograph of the ML projection in figure 32. ▶